Toxic Relief

Don Colbert, M.D.

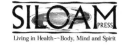

Living in Health—Body, Mind and Spirit

TOXIC RELIEF by Don Colbert, M.D.
Published by Siloam Press
A part of Strang Communications Company
600 Rinehart Road
Lake Mary, Florida 32746
www.siloampress.com

Unless otherwise noted, all Scripture quotations are from the Holy Bible,
New King James Version. Copyright © 1979, 1980, 1982
by Thomas Nelson, Inc., publishers. Used by permission.

Scripture quotations marked KJV are from the King James Version of the Bible.

Scripture quotations marked NIV are from the Holy Bible,
New International Version. Copyright © 1973, 1978, 1984,
International Bible Society. Used by permission.

Cover design by Judith McKittrick

This book is not intended to provide medical advice or to take
the place of medical advice and treatment from your personal physician.
Readers are advised to consult their own doctors or other qualified health
professionals regarding the treatment of their medical problems. Neither
the publisher nor the author takes any responsibility for any possible
consequences from any treatment, action or application of medicine,
supplement, herb or preparation to any person reading or following
the information in this book. If readers are taking prescription
medications, they should consult with their physicians and not take
themselves off of medicines to start supplementation without the
proper supervision of a physician.

Library of Congress Card Number: 2001091178
International Standard Book Number: 0-88419-760-3

02 03 04 05   12 11 10 9 8
Printed in the United States of America

This book is dedicated to Kyle, my teenage son.
Due to the long hours working at my busy medical
practice and the evenings spent researching and writing,
I have been unable to spend adequate time with Kyle.
I want to let Kyle and the whole world know how much I love
him and how I desire and plan to spend more time with
him laughing and having fun.

Acknowledgments

I would like to thank Stephen Strang, publisher of Siloam Press, for allowing me the opportunity of writing this book as well as the many others. I also thank him for having the belief in me to communicate a much needed and timely message.

I would also like to thank Peg de Alminana for her insight, input and organization that went into this book as well as the other publications. I appreciate her sensitivity and the anointing that is on her life.

I wish to thank my wife, Mary, for her much needed love and support during the writing of this book.

Contents

FOREWORD

Don Colbert came to Oral Roberts University in August 1977 as a sophomore. After completing his undergraduate work, he went on to complete medical school at ORU as well. During that time he walked through a life-threatening experience that heightened his awareness of the healing power of God. Because of the supernatural healing he experienced firsthand, Dr. Colbert became a man set on fire to bring God's health and wellness to as many people as humanly possible.

In 1963, ORU was founded on the principle of educating the "whole man"—body, mind and spirit. I knew in my heart that God wanted us to be well in every area of life. God created each of us in perfect balance, and if any part of that balance is out of line, every part suffers. Each person can be treated that way in medicine as well. We are spirit, we live in a body, and we have a mind.

Dr. Colbert is carrying out God's commitment to the whole-man concept. His knowledge of the body being interconnected to the mind and spirit is quite unique. His application of that knowledge helps provide an atmosphere for the whole man to get well. Dr. Colbert believes that by treating all parts as being interrelated, it gives the person a better chance to be brought back into balance in all areas.

This book addresses the whole-man concept in a medical fashion that also includes the necessary awareness of the mind and spirit being treated with equal importance in the body. Because of his many personal experiences in finding health and wellness, God has uniquely gifted Dr. Colbert with an ability to see beyond the sickness and see into the person. He has chronicled that knowledge in this book in order to pass it on to those who desire to search out new answers to age-old problems.

It is my prayer that you too may experience the same wellness that Dr. Colbert and many of his patients have experienced. I thank God for His healing power that is so very important to us all, and I thank God for Dr. Colbert's desire to spread that healing knowledge of the whole man with books such as this one. May God richly bless you as you read.

–ORAL ROBERTS

INTRODUCTION

You need toxic relief. The wealth and privilege of modern America have come at a terrible price. We have created a lifestyle that is so toxic that we've become toxic, too—and it's killing us! Our air is toxic; our water is polluted; our food is depleted of nutrients and packed with poisonous chemicals and hormones; viruses and bacteria are rampant. Not only that, but our minds and hearts often get polluted also.

Someone once told me that if our bodies were sold on the open meat market, they are so full of toxic poisons that they wouldn't pass USDA inspection. I believe it could be true!

We live in a dangerously toxic state, and sadly, most of us aren't even aware of it. Deaths related to our toxic diet and lifestyle account for most deaths in America. Heart disease, cancer, strokes, diabetes, obesity and other diseases cause more than 85 percent of all deaths.[1]

Many diseases are not only related to diet and lifestyle, but they are also caused by a buildup of toxins that have overwhelmed the body's vital organs and other systems, creating an array of distressing symptoms. These include fatigue, memory loss, premature aging, skin disorders, arthritis, hormone imbalances, chronic fatigue, anxiety, emotional disorders, cancers, heart disease and much, much more.

After years as a medical practitioner and family physician, I'm convinced that there's a better way. Yes, we are toxic, and many of us suffer from long lists of chronic illnesses as a result. But we are not hopeless. There is toxic relief!

Much of the pain, suffering and consequential early death caused by our toxic lifestyle can be avoided and even reversed. That's why I've written this book. *Toxic Relief* is a practical book of encouragement and genuine hope. Not only can you prevent chronic illness and poor health due to toxicity, but if you are currently suffering from chronic disease and illness, you may even be able to turn your situation completely around. In this book, I have created a medically sound and easy-to-follow program to give you toxic relief.

With a special diet to get your liver and GI tract in shape, and a program of short, easy juice fasts, together with some lifestyle changes, you really can cleanse your body. By cleansing your system of built-up toxins, you truly will feel better than you have in years.

Deep cleansing your body right down to the cellular level will renew your vitality, restore your energy, reclaim your health, shed toxic fat, lengthen your life and give you a healthy glow you haven't had in years.

Not only that, but this program of fasting and detoxification is also for the total person. Fasting as a spiritual discipline is as old as Moses. This program is designed to cleanse and restore you to health–body, mind and spirit!

So, if you've been suffering from toxic overload of the body, mind and spirit, get ready to experience blessed toxic relief.

–Don Colbert, M.D.

SECTION I—
YOU NEED TOXIC RELIEF

ONE

Our Toxic Earth

The pilot's voice announced our descent into the Los Angeles airport as I looked out the window at the familiar circle of brownish-orange haze surrounding the city of more than three and a half million individuals. In moments we'd descend into that thick cloud of carbon monoxide, lead, ozone, sulfuroxides and nitrogen oxides, and the orange-brown color would vanish from sight. The heavy atmosphere of pollution would soon become indiscernible to the naked eye.

Why? Because as the plane lowered us into that atmosphere, our lungs, hearts, brains, muscles and skin would become additions to that toxic place. We would become part of it—and it would become a part of us.

In a matter of minutes we would rush from the plane to make our various connections, and the ugly brownish-orange ring of pollution would be far from our minds.

As the flight attendants made their final rounds, collecting leftover wrappers and snapping up trays, I wondered how many individuals on that plane were even aware of the long-term health risks to their bodies that simply breathing, eating and living in such pollution cause. No doubt the bodies of everyone around me were already laboring under a heavy toxic burden of which they might be completely unaware. Every human frame was probably in some stage of immune-system breakdown and advancing disease. Some felt fatigued, but couldn't tell why. Others struggled with allergies, arthritis, heart disease, emphysema—some even had cancer.

Sadly, many would never understand that it could have been otherwise.

We live in a toxic world—a toxic planet that is taking a heavy toll upon our bodies every day, whether we know it or not. Due to our technological advances since the Industrial Revolution, we have continued to pour dangerous chemicals and pollutants into our streams, soil and air. At this moment, you probably have some amount of lead in your body, usually stored in your bones—all of us do.[1] Most of us have small amounts of DDT (or its metabolite DDE, which is what it changes into during metabolism) in our fatty tissues.

Existing environmental lead levels are at least five hundred times greater than prehistoric levels.[2] Lead is still one of the most commonly used metals (other than iron), which is used for manufacturing batteries, chemicals and other metal products. Lead has actually contaminated our entire planet. Lead has even been found in some of the most remote areas on the planet such as the Arctic Ice Cap and in the New Guinea aborigines that live far away from any sources of lead exposure. The contamination is most likely due to airborne pollution. It has actually been established that we have between five hundred to seven hundrd times more lead in our bones than our ancestors did.[3]

Unfortunately, much of our water, food and air is polluted by chemicals that are nonbiodegradable, or that take many years to break down. Not only is it difficult for the earth to break down these chemicals, but it is also difficult for your body to detoxify or eliminate them efficiently. Many times we lack the enzymes required to metabolize them. Thus, these chemicals become stored in our bodies, especially in fatty tissues, and are even stored in the brain, which is made of about 60 percent lipids, which are fatlike substances.

SICK AND TOXIC

As a youngster, did you ever take a celery stick and let it sit in a glass of blue or red water overnight? What happened? You woke up the next morning to find a blue or red stick of celery. As the celery took in the water, it turned the color of its environment.

Our bodies are no different. They do not exist separately from the environment in which they live. If our water is polluted, our bodies will become polluted in the same way. If our air is toxic, our lungs will be toxic, too.

If our earth is sick and toxic, then there is a very good chance that most of us will be sick and toxic. Unfortunately, we are usually unable to smell, taste, see or sense most of the toxic chemicals to which we are exposed on a daily basis. As a result, it becomes increasingly difficult to avoid exposure.

Every day we are exposed to thousands of toxins, and they are slowly accumulating in our bodies. If we do not get toxic relief, these poisons may eventually kill us through sickness and disease.

But we are not hopeless. We do not need to sit passively by while our immune systems break down under the heavy burden. Toxic relief is available. You can cleanse your body from years of accumulated toxins and their effects by learning to support your body's own elaborate system of detoxification.

Let's take a closer look at the toxins with which our bodies must deal in an ongoing way.

AWASH IN CHEMICAL CHAOS

Our bodies are battling an onslaught of toxic chemicals of

staggering proportions. Los Angeles is not the only toxic city. In 1993 alone, more than 1,672,127,735 pounds of toxic chemicals were released into our air, according to the Environmental Protection Agency's *Toxic Release Inventory of 1993*.[4]

The air you breathe is polluted by exhaust from our cars, buses, trains and planes, and by industrial air pollution, air pollution from waste disposal and more. Carbon monoxide makes up about half of our air pollutants. Most of this comes from fuel. This dangerous gas has been directly linked to heart disease.[5]

Heavy metals and other pollutants are emitted from smelting plants, oil refineries and incinerators. Ozone is the main chemical offender in smog. It irritates the eyes as well as the respiratory tract. The smog and air pollution in Los Angeles County is so high at times in the summer months that residents are warned against exercising outside. The air can become so thick with chemicals that at times it can be difficult to see.

You can live for weeks without food and days without water, but only minutes without air. If the air you are inhaling contains smog, chemicals, carbon monoxide, heavy metals and other pollutants, then it passes into your nose, into your lungs and on through your bloodstream. With each breath, toxic chemicals are actually being pumped by the heart to every cell in your body via the bloodstream.

Industrial plants, incinerators and hazardous waste sites release volatile organic chemicals. These may include benzene, formaldehyde, vinyl chloride, toluene, carbon tetrachloride and other volatile organic chemicals. Many of these can cause cancer. (See Appendix A.)

INDOOR POLLUTION

If you think that pollution is only found out of doors, you are wrong. Indoor pollution is often even more dangerous to your health than what you inhale outside. Let's look.

Most people spend about 90 percent of their time inside homes, office buildings, restaurants, factories and school buildings. In these places, indoor toxins, chemicals and bacteria get trapped and recirculated throughout the heating and air conditioning systems of these structures, and may create a much greater health risk.

Today's buildings are much more airtight and well insulated than they were years ago, making them vaults for germs, bacteria and chemical toxins. If you travel with your job or business, you could be even worse off. Sealed-tight airplanes can seal in germs, bacteria and pollutants collected from people around the globe.

SICK BUILDING SYNDROME

Think you're safer because your office building is new? I hate to have to be the one to inform you, but you couldn't be more wrong. Volatile organic compounds such as benzene, styrene, carbon tetrachloride and other chemicals are as much as one hundred times greater in new buildings compared to the levels found outdoors.

New buildings are the worst. Building materials emit gasses into the air through a process known as "out-gassing." New carpets release formaldehyde. Paints release solvents such as toluene and formaldehyde, and furniture made from pressed wood releases formaldehyde into the air as well. Additionally, out-gassing may also occur from fabrics, couches, curtains, carpet padding, glues and more.

The many chemicals released through out-gassing from carpets, paints and glues can become so strong that those who work in these buildings can get really ill. When a building's indoor pollution level rises this high, you are more likely to become ill with *sick building syndrome. Sick building syndrome* is defined as "the occurrence of excessive work- or school-related illness among workers or students in buildings of recent construction." With time, however, these toxic levels gradually decrease.

High amounts of volatile organic compounds can also be found in offices. These compounds are emitted from copying machines, laser printers, computers and other office equipment.

Have you been experiencing headaches that get more severe at work? Are your eyes itchy, red and watery? What about a sore throat, dizziness, nausea and problems concentrating? These are just a few of the many symptoms associated with sick building syndrome.

Other symptoms of sick building syndrome include nasal congestion, shortness of breath, problems with memory and concentration, fatigue and itching. In addition, carpet glues as well as particleboard, which is also made from glues and chemicals that contain formaldehyde, commonly cause both fatigue and headaches.

ARE YOU BREATHING IN BACTERIA, MOLD AND YEAST?

Sick building syndrome is not only caused by new materials. Airborne mold, bacteria and the poisons given off by yeast can also cause sick building syndrome. Many people remember the mysterious deaths in 1976 of 182 Legionnaires who were staying at a Philadelphia hotel while attending a conference. It was later determined that this group of people contracted pneumonia from legionella bacteria that had contaminated the hotel's air conditioning system. Before this event, occurrences of sick building syndrome were virtually unheard of.

Nevertheless, many, if not most, air conditioning units and heating systems contain some amount of mold. Significant amounts are frequently found in them, and the spores from that mold can travel throughout a building.

Mold grows wherever dampness is found, which makes air conditioning units incubators for it. Damp homes not only breed mold, but they also breed dust mites. Dust mites are the most common airborne allergy.

PESTICIDE POLLUTION

Dampness is not the only danger to a healthful indoor environment. Dangerous indoor pollution is also created with the ever-increasing use of pesticides, which can be found in some really surprising products.

Believe it or not, pesticides can be found in disposable diapers, shampoos, air fresheners, mattresses and carpets. You are being exposed to pesticides every day. You may even have your home sprayed regularly with pesticides to control bugs.

The most common pesticides in use today are of a variety called *organophosphates*. This group includes diazinon. Pesticides are easily absorbed into your body through contact with your skin, by breathing them into your lungs and by ingesting them through your mouth. Even though your body is designed to eliminate such dangerous poisons, the sheer amount of them that you encounter daily is far more than your body was ever designed to deal with. Therefore, pesticides, their metabolites and other dangerous toxins eventually build up in your body over time. And the greater the buildup, the more difficult it becomes for your body to eliminate them. When such a residue of pesticides builds up in your body, you can begin to experience the following symptoms or diseases:

○ Memory loss

○ Depression

○ Anxiety

○ Psychosis

○ Other forms of mental illness

☼ Parkinson's and other forms of neurological degeneration

☼ Possibly hormone-sensitive cancers such as breast and prostate cancer

ARE YOU BEING FORCED TO INHALE SECONDHAND SMOKE?

Another powerful offender is cigarette smoke. The smoke from a burning cigarette as it sits lit in an ashtray contains a higher toxic concentration of gasses than what the smoker actually inhales.[6]

Secondhand cigarette smoke contains cadmium, cyanide, lead, arsenic, tars, radioactive material, dioxin (which is a toxic pesticide), carbon monoxide, hydrogen cyanide, nitrogen oxides, nicotine, sulfur oxides and about four thousand other chemicals.

Nicotine in the cigarette smoke is the main cause for the cigarette addiction. However, nicotine also constricts blood vessels and stimulates the cardiovascular system and the nervous system. One of the main dangers involved with cigarette smoke is caused by the cancer-causing substances and toxins found in the tars in smoke.

TOXINS IN OUR FOOD AND LAND

Pesticides continue to be sprayed onto our land, subsequently making their way into our food supply. As we eat pesticide-tainted fruits and vegetables, and especially fatty meats, pesticides become stored in our fatty tissues, which not only include our adipose tissue but also the brain, the breasts and the prostate gland.

Every year approximately 1.2 billion pounds of pesticides and herbicides are sprayed on the crops in America that make up our food supply. The farmers who work closely with these chemicals are at a greatly increased risk of developing certain cancers, especially brain cancer, prostate cancer, leukemia and lymphoma. Studies on farmers reveal that as our exposure to pesticides and herbicides is increased, so is our risk for non-Hodgkin's lymphoma.[7]

Some of these dangerous substances are known to last for hundreds and even thousands of years before breaking down.

DDT is an example of a chemical that doesn't break down. It was used in this country on a large scale from the early 1940s to 1972. It is an extremely dangerous poison that was banned in 1972 due to its devastating effect on wildlife, causing multiple abnormalities in the egg shells of many birds and deformities of reproductive organs of many other animals. Bald eagles, condors, alligators and other animals developed deformities and their populations decreased dramatically. Nevertheless, DDT residues are still present in the bodies of practically all Americans. DDT belongs to the class of pesticides known as organochlorines. Many of these have been known to cause cancer and birth defects. They are also stored in the body's fatty tissues.

In 1962, environmentalist Rachel Carson wrote a book called *Silent Spring*, which demonstrated the toxic and deadly effect that DDT has on our food chain.[8]

Carson warned us that if pesticides could have such harmful and dramatic effects on animals and birds, then their effects upon humans would be no different. Nearly forty years ago, this insightful woman actually predicted the global consequences of environmental pollution in her eye-opening book.

Despite the ban of DDT, it still found its way into our soil and our vegetables, especially root vegetables such as potatoes and carrots.

There are over six hundred pesticides used in the United States. However, the Environmental Protection Agency has named sixty-four pesticides as potentially cancer-causing compounds. For more information on pesticides in our food please refer to my book *Walking in Divine Health.*

As I stated before, all of us here in the United States have residues of DDT, or its close relative DDE, in our fatty tissues.[9] Tragically, even though many of these extremely dangerous toxic pesticides were banned for use in the United States, manufacturers are still permitted to export them abroad. We send these poisons to Mexico and other Third World countries for their crops, and then import foods tainted with them back into this country.

Dairy products are one of the main sources of DDT in our diets, and freshwater fish is usually tainted with DDT and PCBs.

Pesticides have been linked to a lower sperm count in men and to higher amounts of xenoestrogen in women. Xenoestrogens are chemical counterfeits that fool the body into accepting them as genuine estrogen. These estrogens are more potent than the estrogen made by the ovaries. When this occurs, a woman's hormones can get way out of balance, leading to symptoms of PMS, fibrocystic breast diseases and potentially endometriosis. It can even have a stimulating effect on breast cancer and endometrial cancer.[10]

WAXES THAT DON'T WASH OFF

No doubt you've tried to wash off a shiny red apple or a dark green cucumber, only to find that it was covered with a layer of waxy film that's nearly impossible to wash off.

Growers do this on purpose. Thick waxes are applied to nearly everything we buy in the produce section of our grocery stores. The wax keeps the produce from dehydrating by sealing in water and also gives vegetables more eye appeal. Fruits and vegetables that have been waxed look bright, shiny and healthy.

Most of these waxes, however, contain powerful pesticides or fungicides that have been added to keep the food from spoiling. These waxes are made to stay on, not wash off. Nevertheless, if you want to stay healthy, remove them.

PESTICIDES IN ANIMAL FEED

Not only can heavy concentrations of pesticides be found in the fruits and vegetables we eat, but they are also in animal feed. Therefore our meat supply ends up tainted with pesticides, too.

Pesticide chemicals accumulate in the fatty tissues of the animals we eat. When we bite into a fatty piece of steak, a greasy hamburger, sausages, bacon or even butter and cream, we are ingesting even more pesticide residues.

TOXIC FAT?

Are you overweight, even a little? Your body is designed to eliminate the toxins you eat. But when pesticides are not broken down and eliminated from your body, they become stored in your fatty tissues. Consider those love handles a hiding place for stored toxins and poisons. In other words, fat is usually toxic, too.

Since your brain is composed of about 60 percent fat, some of these poisons will end up being stored in it as well as in the breasts, prostate gland and any other fatty tissue in the body.

IN THE BRAIN

Many of those suffering with neurological diseases probably have higher levels of pesticides stored in their brains and other fatty tissues.

Have you ever gone on a diet, only to find that you feel more forgetful, foggy-minded and fatigued? When you diet, those pesticides stored in your fatty tissues can be released and may be deposited in the fatty tissue of the brain. You see, often the liver is unable to break down and eliminate adequately the pesticides that have been liberated from your fatty tissues. This can send even more of these residues to the brain as they seek a place to be stored.

IN THE BREASTS

As I mentioned, certain pesticides can pass themselves off in the body for the female hormone estrogen. Therefore, such toxins are called xenoestrogens.

Since high levels of estrogen are linked to breast cancer, high levels of counterfeit estrogens, or xenoestrogens, can also promote cancer. Xenoestrogens mimic estrogen by stimulating estrogen receptors in the body. Therefore, when you ingest increasing levels of certain pesticides, the incidence of breast cancer rises.

For example, a study from Israel showed a decline in the incidence of breast cancer among Israeli women following the enactment of a law against using pesticides.[11]

Here in the United States, we manufacture more than 1.3 billion pounds of pesticides every year. That means each one of us is exposed to pesticides every day. Various types of pesticides can actually act even more powerfully as they are combined with others, dramatically increasing their toxicity.

TOXINS IN OUR WATER

Most chemicals that have been emitted into our air, sprayed on our farmlands or dumped in our landfills will eventually end up in our water. Rains wash these chemicals out of the air and off our land into our lakes and rivers.

Pesticides, herbicides and fertilizers, which contain nitrates, eventually end up in underground aquifers. The toxins gathered in chemical waste sites and dump sites, including landfills, can also eventually seep into our water supplies and contaminate them. Even underground storage tanks that hold gasoline can leak into the ground water.

Rainstorms can actually wash these toxic chemicals into streams and larger bodies of water. Sooner or later, they find their way into our drinking water supply.

The Kellogg Report stated that the growth of industry in this century has been responsible for the introduction of new, complex and sometimes lethal pollutants into our nation's water systems. Municipal treatment plants neither detect nor detoxify the water supply of the majority of chemical pollutants, according to the report.[12]

Undrinkable water is now a major problem in the United States due to chemical pollution. About 50 percent of our underground water, or ground water, is contaminated.

Ground water supplies drinking water for approximately half of the people in America. Often municipalities treat ground water with aluminum to remove organic material, and traces of aluminum remain in the drinking water.

Chlorine is added to the water to kill microorganisms. Chlorine can also combine with organic materials to form trihalomethanes, which are cancer-promoting substances. We increase our risk of developing bladder and rectal cancer by drinking chlorinated water. In fact, the risk increases as our intake of chlorinated water increases.

Trihalomethenes such as chloroform evaporate out of the water during a hot shower and are then inhaled. In fact, a ten-minute hot shower can increase the chloroform absorbed into our bodies more than drinking a half gallon of chlorinated tap water.

Although chlorine kills most bacteria, it does not kill viruses and parasites. Parasites include protozoa such as amoeba, giardia and cryptosporidium. Parasites also include the helminths, which are worms, and arthropods, which are ticks, mites and other bugs. Giardia is one of the major causes of diarrhea in day-care centers. Giardia contaminates many of the lakes and streams in America. You may be drinking them in your own water.

CHEMICAL CHAOS AND WILDLIFE

Pesticides, solvents, industrial chemicals, industrial waste, petroleum products and thousands of other chemicals are already exacting a terrible toll on our wildlife.

Here in Florida where I live, we saw this close up at Lake Apopka, a beautiful body of water I drive by often.

In the book *Our Stolen Future,* Theo Colborn recorded the effects of a pesticide spill that occurred in 1980 in Lake Apopka. Following the spill, the alligator population was studied by a biologist from the University of Florida, along with a biologist from the U. S. Fish and Wildlife Service and the Florida Game and Freshwater Fish Commission. They found that the female alligators' ovaries had abnormalities in both their eggs and egg follicles, similar to what happens in humans who are exposed to DES early in childhood.

The male alligators revealed structural abnormalities as well. Their testes and penises were smaller than normal. In addition, the males also had elevated levels of estrogen and significantly reduced levels of testosterone.[13]

The pesticide spill also affected turtles in Lake Apopka. Researchers found a striking absence of male turtles. They found many female turtles in the lake and many turtles that were neither male nor female, which resulted from a large-scale hormonal disruption due to the pesticide in the lake. The turtles that should have become males ended up being neither male nor female and therefore remained unable to reproduce.[14]

This study has scary implications for more than just wildlife, for if the hormonal disruption of reptiles can create such effects, what might happen to people over the long term? It's certainly worth thinking about.

Nevertheless, if the poisoning of our planet by all these pesticides isn't enough to create alarm, they are not the only environmental toxins your body must battle. Solvents found in cleaners may also contain dangerous poisons as well.

18

THE DANGERS OF SOLVENTS

Solvents, which are chemicals used in cleaning products, are everywhere. Solvents are chemicals that dissolve other materials that otherwise would not be soluble in water.

Solvents can injure your kidneys and liver. They can also depress the elaborate central nervous system of your body.

Like pesticides, solvents are fat-soluble, which simply means that they are likely to be stored in your fatty tissues, including, of course, your brain.

Solvents have the ability to dissolve into the membranes of your cells, especially your fat cells, and accumulate there. Formaldehyde is commonly used as a solvent in many different ways. Manufacturers use it to make drapes, carpet and particleboard—even cosmetics!

Phenol is another common solvent widely found in cleaning products. This dangerous chemical is actually used in making aspirin and sulfa drugs. Phenol is easily absorbed by your skin.

Toluene is another solvent that is similar to benzene. It is used for making a variety of different glues and typewriter correction fluids. If you have elevated levels of toluene in your body, you might experience arrhythmias of the heart as well as nerve damage.

Benzene is a solvent used in making dyes and insecticides. Long-term exposure to benzene can cause leukemia.

The final solvent we are going to look at is vinyl chloride, which is used in the manufacture of PVC pipes and plastic food wrappers. This chemical has been linked to several types of cancers and sarcomas.

Other common toxins include the industrial chemicals PCB, which were banned in 1977. Many lakes and streams are contaminated with PCBs. Increased amounts of PCBs in the body are associated with an increased risk or cancer. A great percentage of people have PCBs in their fatty tissues.

Heavy metals such as mercury, lead, cadmium and arsenic are also commonly stored in our bodies due to our toxic environment.

Not only are we exposed to pesticides and solvents, but our bodies must battle about three thousand different chemical food additives.

FOOD ADDITIVES AND FLAVORINGS

Food additives are a long list of chemical substances that are added to your food for flavor, color, to make it last longer and for a host of other reasons. The largest group of food additives is the flavorings. Most of these flavoring agents are synthetic versions made from chemicals. Another group of food additives includes coloring agents, and most of these are also synthetic chemicals.

This may surprise you, but chemical food additives are usually made from petroleum or coal tar products!

Other food additives include preservatives, bleaching agents, emulsifiers, texturizers, humectants and ripening agents, such as ethylene gas, which is sprayed on bananas to make them ripen faster.

So you can see that even your immune system is being bombarded with toxic chemicals from every direction. You are being exposed to pesticides, food additives, solvents and other chemicals through both your food and environment every day.

If that were not enough, your body must also contend with another entire array of toxins that it produces itself, from within. Let's go to the next chapter and take a look.

TWO

A Toxic Battle Within

I f you lived in a perfect, unspoiled environment with no chemicals or poisons, your body would still produce its own toxins. Just like the engine of a car that creates exhaust as it burns fuel to run, in a much more profoundly complex and wonderful way, your body creates many different toxins in an infinite variety of ways just to function.

In a perfect environment, dealing with your body's internal toxins would be a cinch for your liver and excretory system. But when your liver and GI tract and the organs and tissues of the body are bombarded both from without and within with far more poisons than they were ever designed to handle, it can begin to scream for toxic relief.

Not only does your liver have thousands upon thousands of chemical toxins from everywhere to contend with, your body must deal with its own manufactured toxins. Let's take a look at the toxic battle that rages against your body from within.

THE ANTIBIOTIC ATTACK

Which one of us has not taken antibiotics for a bad case of

bronchitis or a serious infection? Going to the doctor and getting antibiotics today is about as common as eating a peanut butter sandwich. But if you have had repeated bouts of antibiotics, or even a single bout of superantibiotics, then you could be at risk for developing an overgrowth of dangerous intestinal bacteria. Let me explain.

Your intestines are filled with good bacteria, called *lactobacillus acidophilus* and *bifidus,* that prevent the overgrowth of bad bacteria (called *pathogenic bacteria* or *microbes*) in your intestinal tract. When you take antibiotics, many of your body's beneficial bacteria can be killed. Your good bacteria function like a fire wall to keep pathogenic bacteria and yeast in check. So when antibiotics throw off the balance, the bad or pathogenic bacteria may grow like a wildfire, out of control with nothing to slow it down or stop it.

Now your body is in trouble, for bad bacteria may produce endotoxins, which may be as toxic as almost any chemical pesticide or solvent that enters your body from outside.

Overgrowth of bacteria in your small intestines can cause excessive fermentation, just like the fermentation that happens when you leave apple cider outside for too long. This fermentation process creates even more poisons, which are called *indoles, skatols* and *amines.*

THE NIGHTMARE OF CANDIDA

Without antibiotics we'd be in trouble. Infections that might have snuffed out a life a century ago are little more than a nuisance today. But we are just beginning to get a full picture of the toll that the overuse of antibiotics has taken on a generation of users.

Mostly unheard of in centuries past, an epidemic of candida and yeast overgrowth has swept through our nation. When the body's delicate balance of good bacteria and yeast is out of balance, a host of symptoms can result, ranging from relatively minor GI disturbances such as bloating, gas and irritable bowel syndrome to major diseases such as psoriasis, colitis and Crohn's disease.

Just like a biblical plague of locusts that ravaged ancient farmlands, yeast overgrowth causes damage to the intestines like a plague of poison. These toxins produced by yeast are absorbed through your intestines and create devastation no less severe to the inside of your body than the disaster upon the land caused by biblical plagues.

For example, candida albicans release over eighty different poisons into the body. The most toxic substances produced by candida albicans are acetaldehyde and ethanol, which is alcohol.

Acetaldehyde is related to formaldehyde, which is the dangerous solvent found in carpets and pressed wood. Formaldehyde is dangerous enough in the small amounts that you might breathe in, but can you imagine what the effect to your body would be of drinking it? The consequences of having it produced inside your body are disastrous!

Acetaldehyde is also extremely toxic to the brain, even more so than ethanol. It causes memory loss, depression, problems concentrating and severe fatigue.

When you consider the potential danger of having strong, devastating poisons created inside your body, you will recognize that the toxins within can do as much or even more damage than environmental toxins.

You may be thinking, *Whew! I'm glad I don't have candida!* If you don't, I'm glad, too. Nevertheless, that doesn't mean that your body isn't battling a toxic war every single day. With or without candida, your cells are in armed combat.

THE MOLECULAR WARFARE OF FREE RADICALS

While you are going about your daily business, a war is raging inside your body at the molecular level. Free radicals are machine-gunning microscopic shrapnel, injuring your cells throughout the day. Let me explain.

For a moment, picture an atom. It has a nucleus, and it has electrons around it. The nucleus is positively charged, and the electrons are negatively charged. It would look something like the sun with the planets around it.

What happens when someone blows smoke in your face or you are exposed to air pollution or radiation? Or what happens when you ingest alcohol or some other chemical or pesticide? The free radicals created by one of these toxins can pull one of the electrons out of orbit. Thus, massive instability begins at the molecular level—remember these are living, electrically charged cells. When the atom, which is missing an electron, becomes unstable, it begins to grab electrons from other nearby molecules to replace it, causing chain reactions.

These unstable electrons are called *free radicals* because they have been freed or liberated from where they were. The chain reactions caused by liberated electrons can send free radicals spraying through your bloodstream and your body, wreaking great havoc and even possibly setting the stage for cancer, heart disease and a host of other potentially fatal diseases.

Think what would happen if a large crane were driven through the streets of Manhattan with an uncontrolled wrecking ball swinging from side to side. The skyscrapers might not fall, but they would be severely damaged. That's similar to what a free radical can do to your cells.

On a different level, free radicals are also formed during the process of oxidation. For example, when metals are oxidized, rust is produced. When oxidation occurs on painted surfaces, the paint begins to flake off. When you cut an apple in half, it turns brown—that is *oxidation*. It also occurs when meat rots. Our bodies are undergoing oxidative processes every day.

Oxidation is actually caused by free radicals. What happens when you place lemon juice on an exposed slice of an apple? The apple slice doesn't turn brown as rapidly because the antioxidant in lemon blocks the oxidative process—it stops the formation of free radicals.

Each of your body's trillions of cells has a protective wrapping around it made of lipids or "fatty" cell membranes. But free radicals, like wrecking balls, can start ricocheting off the cell membranes—damaging the cell membranes and eventually damaging intracellular structures such as the mitochondria and nucleus.

When wood is burned in a fireplace, smoke is produced. In the body, every cell contains mitochondria that produce energy. The heart muscle cells have a lot of mitochondria because they need a lot of energy, but the fat cells have the fewest mitochondria. Oxygen combines with food in the mitochondria to produce energy. However, in the process of energy production, damaging free-radical forms of oxygen are produced instead of smoke. In other words, when wood is burned, smoke is produced. But in our bodies, when energy is produced, free radicals are formed.

When free radicals begin a chain reaction, they must be stopped quickly. Antioxidants from our diet or supplements and antioxidants produced in our bodies rush to the rescue instantly to quench the free-radical fire of activity. Many free radicals occur with normal metabolic processes in all cells in the body. Internal antioxidants such as superoxide dismutase, glutathione peroxidase and catalase work as antioxidants controlling free-radical production.

But problems occur when the level of free-radical activity gets out of control. When the body is overburdened with free radicals from air pollution, pesticides, cigarette smoke, fried foods and polyunsaturated fats in our diet, then excessive amounts of free radicals ravage our cells. They can actually cause the breakdown of the fats in the cell membranes, ravage the proteins and enzymes and then eventually damage DNA, actually causing mutations. These mutations may result in cancer. Free radicals can also damage the cell membranes so badly that viruses can enter. So you can see, free radicals are bad news!

A WAY OF ESCAPE

At this point you may be feeling a bit overwhelmed by the monumental battle your cells, tissues and organs are being faced with each day. Look in the mirror and see the results of this war: premature aging, sickness, chronic fatigue, arthritis, cancer, heart disease and so much more.

Your body is under an aggressive, ongoing assault against an ever-growing burden of toxins that is probably already causing a heavy toll upon your health–whether or not you even know it. But the good news is that you don't have to sit by passively while your God-given entitlement to good health is stolen right out from under your nose. There is toxic relief!

As I mentioned earlier, your body is designed with an incredible system of defense that keeps you healthy even under extreme circumstances–and you never have to give it a second thought. But when the battle becomes overwhelming, when toxins pile high against you over time, your liver and excretory system become overburdened. They simply cannot keep up.

Nevertheless, you can choose to step in and even the score. By undergoing the program of detoxification outlined in the following chapters, you can cleanse your body from a lifetime of toxins and discover the health and vitality that come with toxic relief. Since the burden of toxins has built up in your body over time, you may have learned to accept the fatigue and general lack of vitality that toxicity causes. You'll simply be amazed at how much better you will feel after freeing your body of its toxic burden.

In my practice, I've encouraged many of my chronically

ill patients to undergo detoxification. The results have been simply astonishing. Heart disease, diabetes, hypertension, arthritis, chronic fatigue and many other serious diseases are being absolutely reversed as my patients cleanse their own bodies from toxins. Later in this book, you'll find a chapter devoted to detoxing for specific diseases.

In addition, if you are overweight, even obese, this program of detoxification has the added benefit of slimming you down. And as you've seen, many of the toxins that are stored in your body get trapped in extra fat. Therefore, your health will improve dramatically once those toxins are removed and not just recirculated to other areas of the body. Not only will you feel better and live longer, you'll look better, too.

YOUR PROGRAM FOR TOXIC RELIEF

Here's an overview of my toxic relief program. Plan to commit about a month to feeling better and looking better:

○ You will start by undergoing a two-week diet to strengthen and support your liver and improve your elimination through the GI tract.

○ Then you will go on a juice fast for two to three days (or longer if monitored by a doctor).

○ You will go back on the special diet for your liver and GI tract for another two weeks.

○ You will begin making lifestyle changes and plan to fast periodically to continue to cleanse and maintain your health.

There you have it! As you go through this program, you will discover renewed energy, rejuvenated health and a fresh, glowing sense of vitality that will absolutely astonish you.

Toxic relief is for your total person. As you learn about this program of toxic relief, you will discover that not only does your body labor under a burden of physical toxins, but also your soul and spirit wage their own battle against toxins on another front. As you read through this book, you will discover that this program of toxic relief addresses your soul and spirit, too. So get ready for a brand-new you—inside and out, body, mind and spirit!

Now that you've seen the truly overwhelming toxic picture, turn with me to begin to find healthful, vital, life-giving toxic relief. But first we must face the terrible truth about the American diet.

THREE

Overnourished While Starving?

A n old proverb says that a man digs his own grave with his fork and knife. It's absolutely true! Today in America, we are one of the most overfed and undernourished societies that ever lived.

FACING THE TERRIBLE TRUTH ABOUT THE AMERICAN DIET

Most of America's health problems today are caused by dietary abuses. Elizabeth Frazao of the U. S. Department of Agriculture reported poor eating habits are linked to more than half of the deaths in the U.S.

Diet is a significant factor in the risk of coronary heart disease (CHD), certain types of cancer, and stroke—the three leading causes of death in the United States, and responsible for over half of all deaths in 1994. Diet also plays a major role in the development of diabetes (the seventh leading cause of death), hypertension, and obesity. These six health conditions incur considerable medical expenses, lost work, disability, and premature deaths—much of it unnecessary, since a significant proportion of these conditions is believed to be preventable through improved diets.[1]

SUGAR ADDICTS

For starters, we're a nation of sugar addicts. The average American consumes 11,250 pounds of sugar during his or her lifetime. That's half a truckload! That means that we're shoveling a small mountain of sugar into our bodies throughout our lifetimes.[2]

PROCESSED FOODS

Processed foods are convenient and inexpensive; for example, white bread, hot dogs, bologna and so on. However, the price you will be paying in the future does not justify the short-term convenience. We really end up robbing Peter to pay Paul.

Processed foods are another method of dietary abuse of our bodies. They generally are so manipulated to prolong shelf life that they are grossly deficient in nutrients. They usually contain food additives, sweeteners, flavorings, coloring agents, preservatives, bleaching agents, emulsifiers, texturizers, humectants, acids, alkalis, buffers and other chemicals. As a result of ingesting processed foods, our tissues and organs must continually draw from our bodies' stored nutrient reserves, setting us up for nutrient deficiencies. No wonder we are overfed with processed foods yet undernourished. Such foods provide loads of calories with little nutrition.

DEAD FOODS

Devitalized food is another way of abusing our bodies instead of nourishing them. When foods have been grown in nutrient-poor soil, they end up looking pretty, but that's about all. When our soil has been robbed of important minerals and nutrients, the food it produces will be nutritionally poor as well.

FAT ABUSERS

The fat we eat, including saturated fats and hydrogenated fats, overtax our bodies with thick sludgelike, yellowish-brown material that encrusts the inside of our arteries, forms plaque, fattens our bodies and shortens our lives. The fats we eat are another dietary abuse against our bodies.

FAST FOODS

Fast foods, fried foods and eating way too much meat while denying our bodies healthful fruits and vegetables are, again, just more ways in which we abuse our bodies through our diets.

GENETICALLY ENGINEERED FOODS

The National Academy of Sciences released a report stating that genetically engineered products introduce new allergens, toxins, disruptive chemicals and unknown protein combinations into our bodies. Pesticidal foods have been grown that are genetically engineered to produce their own pesticide. When we ingest these foods, we will also be ingesting the pesticide produced by the food.

It's too early to tell all the side effects and dangers of these foods. However, we are already seeing the allergic effects. Unfortunately for us in the United States, these foods are not required to be labeled as they are in other countries. However, some manufacturers do label their products as being free of genetically engineered ingredients. Careful shoppers can thus avoid genetically engineered foods.[3]

It's easy to see why we're overfed and undernourished. We gorge ourselves with increasing amounts of food to respond to our bodies' cravings for nutrition. After we've eaten, our bodies, even though under a heavy burden of calories, still realize that they never received the nutrients they needed. So our brains send more signals, triggering hunger, which is interpreted by us as the need or desire for even more food. We end up spiraling down into a vicious cycle of overfeeding with empty foods, craving more nutrition and overfeeding again with even more empty processed, devitalized, sugary foods.

The end result is ever-expanding waistlines, thighs and buttocks. We get fatter and fatter, forcing our bodies to groan under the burden of extra pounds. But in terms of actual nourishment, we give our bodies less and less.

OBESE WHILE STARVING?

We may be actually starving from a nutritional standpoint, while at the same time becoming grossly obese. The end result of this merciless abuse of our bodies is disease and death. Sadly, we really are digging our graves with our forks and knives!

As a result of our overindulgences we have an epidemic of heart disease, atherosclerosis, hypertension, diabetes, cancer, allergies, obesity, arthritis, osteoporosis and a host of other painful and debilitating degenerative diseases.

EATING TOO MUCH OF THE WRONG STUFF?

Many people have the mistaken notion that they can exist on junk food day by day and then take a multivitamin or a multitude of vitamins a day and still maintain excellent health. Some people even do this trying to reverse degenerative diseases. Unfortunately, many doctors and nutritionists are pushing this fallacy, often out of ignorance.

Taking vitamins and other nutrients and continuing to eat poorly is similar to never changing the oil or oil filter in your car and yet continuing to drive it. Periodically you might add small amounts of oil to the car to keep the oil level in normal range. This is, in essence, what most people are doing in their mistaken belief that they can continue to eat junk food, yet take a vitamin a day or multitudes of vitamins and be healthy.

I've had patients who have brought in very large suitcases filled with supplements of all kinds. Unfortunately, these have been some of my sickest patients. That's because they continued to eat whatever they pleased, foolishly believing that supplements alone could make up for whatever their diet was lacking.

How wrong they were! Some were literally spending thousands of dollars every month and getting sicker by the day.

Most chronic diseases, such as heart disease, diabetes, arthritis and cancer, are usually associated with nutritional deficiencies. However, dieting and too much sugar, fats, processed foods, fast foods and other devitalized foods are literally draining the life out of us as they constipate our bodies, introduce toxins and drain us of our nutrient reserves. Americans have been duped into believing that we can continue to eat whatever we want and that simply taking a vitamin or a multitude of vitamins can neutralize or protect ourselves from whatever we have eaten.

UNDERNOURISHMENT AND DISEASE

When treating those with degenerative diseases, I began to notice a pattern. Most of these individuals weren't underfed. In fact, most of them were big overeaters. They ate plenty—but they ate all the wrong things. They were overfed and yet completely undernourished.

This was particularly true of people with obesity, cardiovascular diseases, arthritis, Type 2 diabetes, migraine headaches, a host of different allergic conditions, psoriasis, rheumatoid arthritis and lupus. In fact, to some degree, it appeared to apply to nearly all degenerative diseases.

For many of these people, medications won't help. Nor can taking vitamins and nutrients eliminate the cause of these diseases. That's because it's not lack that causes many of these diseases—it's eating too much.

I began to realize that one of the main causes of these degenerative diseases is overconsumption of sugary, fatty, starchy and high-protein foods—foods that have been processed, fried and further devitalized. These people were taking in enormous amounts of empty, fattening calories, but they were not nourishing their bodies.

Taking some supplements such as a comprehensive multivitamin with minerals, antioxidants and so forth is important. However, much more important are eliminating or significantly reducing consumption of the fats, sugars, processed "dead" foods and eating more fruits, vegetables, whole grains, nuts, seeds and other "living" foods.

Taking in dead, nonbeneficial food creates a trap. When your body realizes that it hasn't received the nourishment it craves, even after you've eaten a large, calorie-laden meal, your brain sends a signal that it still needs nourishment. But when you answer that craving with more dead food, you start a cycle that leaves your body laboring under a devastating burden of too much sugar, starch and fat and not enough nourishment.

This kind of burden creates enormous stress for your entire digestive tract. It overtaxes the liver and overwhelms your entire body with massive amounts of dangerous fats, chemicals and other toxins.

All the while, in a sense you are starving. You are becoming depleted of what you really need: essential vitamins, minerals and antioxidants. Eating in this way will make you feel fatigued and irritable, and over time you'll begin to develop one or more of the degenerative diseases listed above.

Overnutrition is worse than undernutrition. In fact, animal studies have shown that getting too few calories, which is technically called *calorie restriction,* can actually increase longevity.[4] Although I do recommend calorie restriction for some diseases, such as Type 2 diabetes and obesity, I believe that as a nation we need to work harder at eating in a way that keeps us within a healthy weight range.

WHY CONVENTIONAL MEDICINE CAN'T HELP

Conventional medicine with its prescriptions many times cannot help. Medical specialists will have to address the root of this problem. Thomas A. Edison said, "The doctor of the future will give no medicine, but will interest his patients in the care of the human frame, in diet and in the cause and prevention of disease."[5] What we need is better prevention.

STOP AND THINK ABOUT HOW WE EAT

Our prosperity as a nation has come at a price. After years of overeating and overindulgence, we are experiencing an epidemic of degenerative diseases.

Most of us eat a standard American diet. That means lots of fat, sugar and highly refined wheat products, including white bread, crackers, bagels, pasta and cereals. Add other processed food, such as potato chips, corn chips and white rice. Don't forget the fatty meats like T-bone steaks, ribs, bacon and pork chops. Now, top it all off with a large amount of saturated fat, hydrogenated fat and processed vegetable fat, such as salad dressing, peanut butter, most cooking oils and mayonnaise. It's no wonder we have an epidemic of heart disease, cancer, diabetes and arthritis as well as many other degenerative diseases.

Now for dessert. What could be more American than apple pie? Nevertheless, the absolute worst foods—and all-time American favorites—contain tons of sugar and hydrogenated fat. These include many baked goods, such as cupcakes, cookies, pies, Danishes, fudge and brownies—and don't forget the doughnuts and candy bars.

We didn't always eat this way. Former generations were some of the healthiest on the planet. As an agrarian culture, many of our grandparents lived much closer to the land. But today, our lifestyle is much too stressed and fast-paced, and as a result our diet suffers.

STRESSED OUT?

Most of us are nearly drowning in stress. We live on the run, tossing down dinner from drive-throughs on our way to meetings or our children's activities. On other days, we wash ashore at the end of the day with barely enough strength to make TV dinners. Or worse yet, we fill up on chips or whatever else we can find on the run.

We wear ourselves out working longer hours, and we enjoy our lives less and less. We exercise very little, if at all, and we keep up our hectic pace through stimulants such as coffee, tea, sodas and chocolate. We stress our bodies even more by purchasing more "things," bigger houses and new cars, which means longer work hours to pay for our cravings. Our list of commitments grows while our endurance runs out.

Stressed-out America is on a path to degenerative disease and premature death. Many of us are dying in middle age. But it doesn't have to be this way. We can choose to relax, slow down, smell the roses and choose a healthy diet.

CHANGE THE WAY YOU THINK

Most of us have grown up eating the American diet and feeling pretty good about it. But to live healthier, longer lives, we must rethink what we've been taught about food—before it's too late.

How do we change our thinking? We can start by changing the *why* of eating. Just why do you eat? Do you eat because something tastes good and your flesh is craving it? Or do you eat because you are providing your body with fuel to run? For most Americans, eating has become more of a recreation than a daily necessity based upon nutritional wisdom.

Now, I'm not trying to suggest that eating shouldn't be enjoyed. God created all things for us to enjoy, and eating was one of those things. But when our dietary choices, which were designed to nourish and sustain our bodies, actually begin to make us ill, then we must change the way we think.

Hippocrates, the father of medicine, said, "Our food should be our medicine and our medicine should be our food." In other words, what we eat should be so good for us that it actually heals and restores our bodies. What a difference from the average American mind-set about eating!

Start thinking about more than just taste and pleasure when you eat. Begin to eat for your health's sake!

So, here's your new set of priorities: health first, taste and pleasure second. I guarantee that once you begin to satisfy *the true* need of your body—the need for genuine nourishment—you'll begin to enjoy your food much more.

HEALTH-FIRST EATING

A health-first eating lifestyle begins by eliminating or drastically reducing how much fried food, processed foods, processed vegetable fats, saturated fats, hydrogenated and partially hydrogenated fats and sugar you take in. It also means avoiding fatty cuts of meats and selecting smaller portions of the leanest meats. These include free-range chicken or turkey breast and free-range beef such as extra lean ground round, tenderloin and filet.

FIVE ALIVE

Eat three to five servings (no fewer than three) of living, organic vegetables and two to four servings of fruit every day. That means fruits and vegetables should make up a large percentage of your diet. This is the recommendation of the United States Department of Agriculture, and mine also.

I did my internship and residency training at Florida Hospital, which is run by the Seventh-Day Adventist church. The Seventh-Day Adventists avoid alcohol, tobacco, caffeine and pork. They are also taught to refrain from eating eggs, meats and even fish. Many are strict vegetarians. While I was there as a resident, the cafeteria served vegetarian foods only. Adventists who are vegetarians live about thirteen years longer than the average nonsmoking American.[6]

One such Seventh-Day Adventist was the physician Dr. John Harvey Kellogg. He was a vegetarian who, together with his brother, built a factory in Battle Creek, Michigan, to produce various health foods, including whole-grain cereals. That's where your box of *Special K* comes from. However, Dr. Kellogg didn't process his cereals as the majority are processed today to extend shelf life. Dr. Kellogg believed that 90 percent of all diseases were caused by improperly functioning colons.[7]

One of Dr. Kellogg's patients, C. W. Post, was also an employee. He later developed Post Cereals.[8]

LIMIT MEATS

The Bible does not recommend vegetarianism, so neither do I. Adam and Eve were vegetarians in the Garden of Eden, and some prophets, such as John the Baptist, Samson and others who had taken Nazirite vows, were vegetarians. Still, Jesus Christ was not.

Nevertheless, most Americans eat far too much meat. I recommend that women eat only 2 to 3 ounces of lean, free-range meat, preferably only once daily, or at the most twice daily. Men, limit meats to only 4 ounces of lean, free-range meat, only one or, at the most, two times a day.

If you have a severe degenerative disease, such as cancer, severe coronary artery disease, rheumatoid arthritis or lupus, then eliminate meats and dairy products entirely or at least until your condition improves significantly.

AVOID HIGH-PROTEIN DIETS

More and more people are going on high-protein diets such as the Atkin's Diet. Yes, they are losing weight. But the long-term effects of this diet can be very dangerous and may lead to many degenerative diseases.

If you are on this diet, limit your protein portions to less than 4 ounces for men and less than 3 ounces for women once or twice a day. For more information on this subject, refer to my book *What You Don't Know May Be Killing You.*

IN CONCLUSION

If you see yourself in this chapter, be encouraged. Even if you've spent a lifetime digging your own grave with your fork and knife, it's never too late to change. You will make many choices about your destiny by what you choose to eat. Choose now to reap health, happiness and a long life. You hold the key to your own future health.

Let's turn now and look at what I believe is the single most effective answer to overnourishment—fasting! More than anything else, fasting is a dynamic key to cleansing your body from a lifetime collection of toxins, reversing overnourishment and the diseases it brings and ensuring a wonderful future of renewed energy, vitality, longevity and blessed health.

SECTION II—
DR. C'S
PROGRAM FOR
DETOXIFICATION

FOUR

Toxic Relief Through Fasting

D avid,* a man who had worked for many years as an environmental engineer, seemed frightened and agitated as he walked into my office. His skin was pallid and deathly gray. His eyes seemed lifeless, and his demeanor was halting and somewhat confused.

He sat down and crossed his arms in disgust after he threw some paperwork on my desk. Visibly shaken, he declared loudly, "My body is more polluted than a toxic waste dump!" He pointed to the shocking results of the hair analysis for heavy metals he had brought with him. "I guess I'm just a walking toxic waste dump. According to these numbers, if my body was a piece of earth, it would be too toxic for my neighbors to live next to!"

The figures didn't lie. If a piece of land contained the toxins that this man's body contained, the government would probably have declared it a toxic waste site. How frightening!

This polluted planet is having a devastating impact upon us. If, like David, we've gotten to the place where our good health and mental acuity are already compromised, then we've almost gone too far.

---

*Fictionalized character created from a composite of accounts

David's eyes filled with fear as he pleaded, "I don't know what to do. I feel awful. I'm tired all the time. I can hardly remember the normal daily details of my life. I expect I'll die of cancer or something worse if this can't be turned around. Can you help me, Doc?"

Although my heart really went out to him, I knew that what David needed was not sympathy. Pure and simple, David needed toxic relief.

What about you? Your body may not be as toxic as David's, but it's still probably a lot more toxic than you might imagine. The good news is that toxic relief is available!

WHAT'S YOUR BODY TRYING TO TELL YOU?

For starters, ask yourself this question: Are you listening to your body? Do you understand what it's trying to tell you?

Sickness and degenerative disease are usually simply nature's way of telling you that your body is toxic and needs to be cleansed. If you were driving your car and the red engine light came on indicating that it was time to check the engine, would you continue to drive the car without taking it to the shop to have it checked? This actually happened to a patient. She ended up having to replace her engine because she ignored the red engine light.

You may laugh, as her family members did when she told me the story. However, this is exactly what many of us are doing. Our red engine light is flashing through the symptoms and signs of degenerative diseases that we are experiencing—diabetes, heart disease, arthritis, headaches, allergies, psoriasis, rheumatoid arthritis, lupus and other degenerative diseases.

Too often we simply ignore the signs and symptoms and continue eating the wrong foods. We also keep living our stressed-out, unhealthy lifestyles of cigarette smoking, drinking alcohol and not exercising.

Our bodies simply weren't designed to handle it all. Nevertheless, we continue to push and stress our bodies with these toxic burdens until they eventually develop diseases. At that point, we then run to the doctor and get medication, which further strains the liver's ability to detoxify and does nothing to cleanse it.

If this sounds like you, chances are you are simply toxic and probably overfed. As I mentioned earlier, simply beefing up your intake of supplements usually won't help. So what can you do?

FINDING RELIEF THROUGH FASTING

The answer is fasting. Fasting is a powerful, natural way to cleanse your body from the burden of excess toxic nutrients, such as bad fats, and from all other chemicals and toxins that cause degenerative diseases.

Fasting is the safest and best way to heal the body from degenerative diseases caused by being overfed with the wrong nutrition.

The ancient father of medicine, Hippocrates, said, "Everything in excess is opposed by nature." Many years as a practicing medical doctor have convinced me that he was right. Our nation is suffering an epidemic of degenerative diseases and death that is caused by excess—plain and simple. We have eaten too much sugar, too much fat, too many empty calories and far too much processed, devitalized food.

PERIODIC FASTING

Finding toxic relief through fasting can turn your life and health around. It is a natural, biblical system of supporting and cleansing the body from built-up chemicals, fats and other toxins. It also has amazing spiritual benefits, as we will see later on.

Periodic fasting, followed by a cleansing diet, will allow you to live free of the physical and neurological burden of toxins. Fasting gives your toxic, overtaxed body an opportunity to "catch up" with its overwhelming task of waste removal.

FASTING—A NATURAL PRINCIPLE OF HEALING

Fasting allows your body to heal by giving it a rest. All living things need to rest, including you. Even the land must rest, which was a principle God gave to the ancient agrarian Jewish nation regarding their fields. Every seventh year they were not permitted to grow any crops at all. They had to let the land lie fallow so that it could reestablish its own mineral and nutrient content. (See Leviticus 25:1–7.)

Today, we live in a time in which farmers have completely forgotten this age-old principle. This is one of the factors involved in our being overfed and undernourished. It's because much of our soil is depleted that our food sources have also become partially depleted of the minerals, vitamins and other nutrients that our bodies crave. When we eat and don't get the nutrition we need from our food, we will usually eat more, trying to fill the body's craving for nourishment. Before long, we have become obese, overfed and undernourished.

Every winter many animals will hibernate or rest for a season. Every night when you sleep, you give rest to your body and mind. Blessed rest is as much a law of the universe as gravity. It's also a powerful principle of healing.

Think about it: When an animal is injured or sick, what does it do? It finds a resting place where it can lap up water, and it quits eating while it heals. This is natural, instinctual wisdom that God placed within the animal kingdom.

But when our bodies get sick, what do we do?

When we get sick with an injury or illness, such as pneumonia, a sinus infection or strep throat, instead of resting and fasting by drinking water or juices only, we eat ice cream, puddings, creamy soups and other rich, high-caloric foods that do nothing to cleanse and detoxify the body.

We also prolong our illnesses by taking Tylenol to suppress the fever so that we can go back to work far sooner than our bodies are ready. We push ourselves by taking antibiotics, decongestants and antihistamines to dry up the mucus. This also impedes the natural process of detoxification. Instead of healing, our bodies may store even more toxic material.

Now I do recommend antibiotics for infectious diseases when they are warranted. Such times include for bacterial infections such as pneumonia, acute bronchitis, urinary tract infections, strep tonsillitis and many other bacterial infections. However, too many doctors prescribe antibiotics for viral infections, allergic symptoms or when a patient requests them. Sometimes they are given because a doctor is unable to figure out what is going on or what is causing the fever.

Hippocrates' saying, "Let your medicine be your food and let your food be your medicine," applies here as well. In other words, let what you take into your body provide healing. Rest the body. Drink plenty of fluids. Drink fresh juices that allow the body to heal. Don't you think humans should have as much sense as the animals?

Hippocrates practiced around 400 B.C. and commonly used medicinal foods such as apples, barley and dates to treat his patients. Aristotle, Plato, Socrates, Galen and Paracelsus all believed in fasting and practiced this therapy. They used fasting, juices, soups, nutrition and rest to bring their patients back to health. Hippocrates treated the patient and not the disease.

GENERAL BENEFITS TO FASTING

Fasting gives a rest to the digestive tract. Your body uses a significant amount of your energy every day in digesting, absorbing and assimilating your food. Since fresh juices are very easy for the body to assimilate, they give your digestive tract a chance to rest and repair. This, in turn, gives your overburdened liver a chance to catch up on its work of detoxification.

Juice fasting, as we will see later, also creates an alkaline environment for your body's cells and tissues so that they can start releasing waste products through your body's various channels of elimination. The primary elimination channels of the body include the kidneys and urinary tract, the colon, the lungs and the skin. Fasting allows your liver to catch up on its internal cleansing and detoxification. At the same time, the digestive organs, including the stomach, pancreas, intestines and gallbladder, get a much deserved rest.

Even the blood and the lymphatic system can be effectively cleansed of toxic buildup through fasting. During fasting, our cells, tissues and organs can begin to dump out accumulated waste products of cellular metabolism as well as chemicals and other toxins. This helps your cells to heal, repair and be strengthened.

You have about sixty to one hundred trillion cells in your body, and each one takes in nutrients and produces waste products. Fasting allows each cell to dump its waste products and thus be able to function at peak efficiency.

Fatty tissues release chemicals and toxins during fasting. These, in turn, are broken down by the liver, excreted by the kidneys and through the bile. Your body will excrete toxins in many different ways during fasting. Some people actually develop boils, rashes or body odor during fasting since toxins are being released through the body's largest excretory organ, the skin.

FASTING ENERGIZES CELLS

Fasting is also an energy booster. The toxic buildup in the cells congests the mitochondria (the energy factories in each cell) so they cannot effectively produce energy. This leads to fatigue, irritability and lethargy. Let me explain. Mitochondria are sites within each of your cells where energy is produced. Metabolic waste, chemicals and other toxins affect the function of the mitochondria of the cell, making them less efficient in producing energy.

REJUVENATE PHYSICALLY, MENTALLY AND SPIRITUALLY

Periodic, short-term fasting will also strengthen your immune system and help you live longer.

Deep cleansing of every cell in your body through fasting has the wonderful added benefit of improving your appearance. As your body detoxifies, your skin will eventually become clearer and glow with a radiance that you probably haven't seen for quite a few years. The whites of your eyes usually become clearer and whiter and may even sparkle.

As toxic fat melts away through fasting, you'll feel and look better than you have in years. Your energy will be supercharged. And your mental functioning usually improves as your body cleanses, repairs and rejuvenates.

Fasting cleanses and rejuvenates the body physically, mentally and spiritually. It is also one of the best ways of preventing and treating sickness and disease, as we will see later.

A CELLULAR GARBAGE DUMP?

Have you ever driven by a garbage dump in the middle of the summer? It isn't a pleasant experience. So, don't let your body become a cellular garbage dump filled with toxins that create degenerative diseases. Instead, cleanse your body periodically with fasting to both prevent or to treat degenerative diseases.

You may be thinking, *Fasting is something that I just cannot do! Fasting is for far more disciplined people than me. It's impossible for me to fast.*

If you've responded this way, you probably see fasting as a feat of unflinching self-denial and other-worldly determination for which only a few are cut out. Certainly not yourself! However, that's simply not true. Although some fasting is little more than a rigorous test of self-endurance, that's not at all the kind of fasting I'm suggesting here.

The detox fast that I will be outlining in the following chapters is not a grueling feat of self-denial. If you carefully follow the steps that I will outline, you will not find fasting difficult at all.

So, let's take a look at the first step, which is the preparation.

LET'S TALK ABOUT FASTING

Fasting in general is very controversial. Many methods of fasting exist, as well as many attitudes about fasting. As a doctor, I've been able to look closely at the various popular methods of fasting. Some of them are good, while others can be downright dangerous. So, before you decide to begin fasting, let's investigate fasting and look carefully at the method of fasting that I'm convinced will put you on a path to healthier living.

FASTING—WHAT IS IT ALL ABOUT?

Despite the fact that many believe that the only true method of fasting is the total fast–not eating or drinking anything–I consider this method to be unsafe. Let's look.

TOTAL FASTING

Fasting is often thought of as taking nothing by mouth. Technically speaking, this is true fasting. But it's not the type of fasting I'm suggesting here for detoxification.

I never recommend total fasting. Your body must always have at least two quarts of water a day to sustain your life, for you can only live for a few days without water.

The kind of fasting that most of us are familiar with is avoiding all solid food and consuming liquids only.

A WATER-ONLY FAST

The strictest, most severe fast is a water-only fast. In general, I usually don't recommend this type of fasting. But for certain autoimmune diseases such as lupus and rheumatoid arthritis or for severe atherosclerosis such as severe coronary artery disease, the benefits of water-only fasting are powerful. Nevertheless, you can also experience similar benefits for these diseases with juice fasting—it just takes longer.

If you are considering water-only fasting, be prepared to completely devote several days to doing little more than fasting. For most individuals, water-only fasting so weakens the body that working a full-time job while fasting is not possible.

If you do not have one of these diseases, I believe that the best fasting method for cleansing and detoxification is juice fasting. Juice fasting provides most of the benefits of water-only fasting without the unpleasant weakness and hunger that often accompany a water-only fast.

JUICE FASTING

The fasting method I recommend for complete detoxification is juice fasting. For this type of fast, you will need lots of fresh fruits, vegetables and a juicer.

Some feel that juice fasting is not really fasting in the truest sense of the word. Others doubt that it has the same benefits of water fasting. And while water-only fasting does have some truly restorative healthful effects, juice fasting can be even more beneficial, and it is far less strenuous, since it supports detoxification, alkalinizes the body and supports the liver. One usually doesn't experience the weakness or hunger of water fasting, and usually experiences tremendous energy during the fast.

As I mentioned, water-only fasting can reduce inflammation in the body. In addition, it may actually cause the hardened arterial plaque of severe coronary disease to regress and possibly melt away. Juice fasting can produce a similar effect, but over an extended period of time.

In addition, raw, freshly squeezed juices supply generous amounts of vitamins, minerals, antioxidants, enzymes and phytonutrients that help your body to restore itself and heal.

Let's take a look at some of the special benefits of juice fasting.

RESTORING NATURE'S DELICATE BALANCE

Few people ever consider that the health of their bodies is based upon a delicate natural acid and alkaline balance. Nevertheless, this balance is essential to your body's ability to detoxify successfully. When all your body gets is the standard American diet, your tissues become more acidic than nature intended—upsetting this delicate balance.

If you'd like to know how acidic your body is, you can find out very easily by simply purchasing some pH strips at the drugstore. Collect the first morning urine and dip a pH paper into it. It will indicate your urine's pH level with a change of color. The urinary pH usually indicates the pH of the tissues. The change of color can then be matched to a numerical reading. A card is included in the pH paper that correlates a color to a pH number.

Most people will have a pH test reading of about 5.0, which means their bodies are very acidic. It should be between 6.8 to 7.0. Close enough doesn't count. Even though five is only two points less than seven, a pH of 5.0 is actually a hundred times more acidic than a pH of 7.0.

CELLULAR CONSTIPATION?

What happens when your body is too acidic? Precious minerals are lost in the urine and cells become less permeable, which means they are unable to excrete waste products effectively. In a sense, your cells become constipated, or each one of them may become full of waste that it cannot get rid of.

When this occurs, the mitochondria or energy-producing structures in the cell do not function properly, and you usually feel fatigued. Your cells become toxic. Now, free-radical activity increases, and the toxic overload just continues to build until your body begins to deteriorate and degenerative diseases occur.

Juice fasting brings back the natural balance. It alkalinizes the tissues and raises the pH. Now the cells can begin to excrete toxins again. Detoxification has begun.

GIVING YOUR GUT A REST

An occasional juice fast—every one, three or six months—gives your gastrointestinal system a much needed rest.

Juices are easy on the digestive system. They are easily absorbed into the body without requiring much work from your stomach and intestines. Water fasts also give the digestive system a rest.

JUICE VS. WATER ONLY

Fasting is not new. As a matter of fact, it's been around since before Moses. Many people go on water-only fasts and believe that this is the only true way to fast. However, this program of juice fasting will usually provide you with more benefits than water fasting, but without many of the drawbacks. Let's take a look.

MUSCLE LOSS

The right kind of juice fast will continue to nourish your body. You won't experience the kind of muscle loss that can happen during a water-only fast. If you're a fan of the television series *Survivor,* you've watched the participants wither away every week, losing large quantities of muscle mass. In essence, except for a few spoons of rice each day, they usually are on a water-only fast. Periodic juice fasting provides the body with so much nutrition that such muscle loss would be minimal.

In addition, prepared correctly, juice can provide the nutrients, amino acids and fuel that your liver requires to detoxify. This is an extremely important aspect of detoxification that we will examine in-depth later on.

Antioxidants

That's not all! Juice fasting has even more cleansing benefits. Correctly prepared, juice can supply a vast array of antioxidants—which you will need to protect your liver from the enormous spray of free radicals that are released during fasting. Water-only fasts decrease the stores of antioxidants, increasing your risk for oxidative damage from free radicals to tissues and organs throughout your body.

Water fasting, and even long-term juice fasting, depletes your body of glutathione. That may not seem that important, but it really is. Glutathione is probably the most important and the most abundant antioxidant in the body. It protects us from free-radical activity and regenerates vitamins C and E. The overworked liver is a hotbed of free-radical activity, and adequate levels of glutathione are essential or the liver can be damaged by free radicals.

To effectively cleanse your body, I believe it is much healthier to go on a series of short juice fasts rather than one long fast. This allows your body time to recuperate and rebuild its stores of antioxidants as well as glutathione.

Healing

Fasting with the right kinds of raw, fresh juices increases the healing benefits of fasting.

Specially prepared juices are packed full of nutrients, phytonutrients and enzymes. These can supply the raw materials your body needs to repair your cells, heal your organs and protect your tissues from free radicals.

JUICE FASTING AND WEIGHT LOSS

This sensible, medically sound method of fasting can very quickly allow you to shed any extra toxic fat that your body may be carrying—even if you're significantly overweight. In addition, you can avoid a water-only fasting trap of which many people are not even aware. What's the trap? Water-only fasting can actually cause you *to gain* significant amounts of weight after the fast!

That's one of the reasons that fasting with a program of specially prepared juices is so much more sensible. Not only that, but it's also much easier to stay on a specially prepared juice fast because your body will not crave nutrition in the same way that it does during a water-only fast.

No METABOLICALLY INDUCED WEIGHT GAIN

The reason for this is because fasting with specially prepared juices does not throw your body into a state of muscle catabolism, which is excessive muscle breakdown.

During a water fast, the body goes into this state and burns muscle tissue as fuel. After about two to three days of burning muscle, which is converted to glucose, as fuel, the body shifts to burning ketones from the breakdown of fat as fuel. Thus after a few days of water fasting, the body begins breaking down more fat and less muscle. Ketosis develops, and the body can become more acidic.

The metabolic rate also slows down. This metabolic slow-down can actually cause you to gain weight after the water fast when you begin to eat again.

Let me explain. When you go on a water-only fast, mechanisms in your brain signal your body that you are starving even if you are not. Therefore, your body goes into a survival state to try and hold onto all of the calories it gets. In this state, you can actually eat nothing and lose only a small amount of weight.

However, your body doesn't immediately move back out

of that state when you start eating again. It may take months for the metabolic rate to recover. Thus when you go back to eating a normal diet, you will usually gain weight rapidly and will often gain more weight. When you do another fast, the metabolic rate may have never fully recoverd, and therefore you may continue to gain more weight after the fast is broken.

This should not happen to you on my specially prepared juice fast. Fasting with the juice program that I have provided in this book will provide your body with enough calories and nutrition so that you should be able to bypass this experience altogether.

The final effect for you will be—weight loss! Not only will this special fasting method free your body of disease-causing chemicals, but it will also free it of toxic fat. If you are over-weight, and even significantly obese, one of the truly wonderful and healthful benefits of this fasting method is that it can help bring your body back to the normal, healthy size that God intended. A regular, sensible fasting program can slim you down very quickly, and you will also experience the more important benefit of eliminating the fatty areas in your body where dangerous toxins and chemicals were stored. Without these stored fatty areas, toxins will have no place to hide and will be detoxified and flushed more readily from your body.

Not only will you live longer through this juice detoxification plan, but you will feel better and look better also!

STAY ENERGIZED

Many fasting programs are so physically challenging that you can be left feeling completely wiped out with little or no energy to function. This juice-fasting program is designed to keep you energized enough to work, play and enjoy your daily activities.

As a matter of fact, since juice fasting will increase both

the detoxification capabilities of the body and increase the elimination of toxins, you may actually experience more energy during this fast, not less.

Liver friendly

Water-only fasting can place considerable additional strain upon an already overworked liver. And since your liver is the primary detoxification organ, you need to do all that you can to support its vital function in your body.

Juice fasting does this, while on the other hand, water fasting usually places more strain on the liver and depletes the liver of glutathione. That's one of the reasons for the overwhelming sense of fatigue you can experience during a water-only fast.

During a water-only fast, a flood of toxins is released from fat and other cells and tissues so quickly that the liver can become overwhelmed trying to keep up the process of detoxification. Such a burden is placed upon the liver at this point that it usually requires more vitamins, minerals, amino acids and antioxidants. Juice fasting supplies the vitamins, minerals, amino acids and antioxidants, but water fasting does not. In addition, a shower of free radicals is created in this flood of released toxins, creating a hotbed of free-radical activity in the liver and possibly injuring the liver.

KEEPING THE COLON IN THE GAME

One of my main concerns about water-only fasting is that it knocks out a major player in the detoxification game—the colon. When you fast with water only, your colon usually shuts down. In a less toxic world, this probably wouldn't matter so much. But with the toxic load with which our bodies are dealing, we don't want this vital detox player sitting on the bench.

One extremely important reason for keeping this vital player in the detox game is DDT, as well as other pesticides. As mentioned earlier, most of us have DDT or DDE (the toxic metabolite of DDT) in our fatty tissues. During a water-only fast in which the colon rests, DDT as well as other pesticides and solvents are released from the fatty tissues into the bloodstream at an extremely rapid rate. This, in turn, can overwhelm the liver so that it cannot detoxify the chemical effectively. If this happens, DDT and other pesticides and solvents can end up in other fatty tissue in the body, including the brain, spinal cord and peripheral nerves.

That's why it's absolutely essential to keep this powerful detox player in the game. Even while you're on this program of juice fasting, you should drink herbal teas to keep the colon functioning. If your colon stops, be prepared to use an herbal tea or a mild enema. We'll discuss more about this later.

IN CONCLUSION

Controversy will always remain between water-fasting and juice-fasting methods. That's why it's important to carefully consider both methods and determine which one will be most effective for you.

Now let's look at juice fasting and the promise it holds for your renewed health and vitality.

FIVE

The Joy of Juice

Recently while traveling in another city, my wife, Mary, was standing at a Clinique counter at a department store and struck up a friendly conversation with a couple next to her in line. The middle-aged man shared that six months previous he had undergone a month-long juice fast. Interestingly, he hadn't fasted at the advice of a medical person or because he had read about it. He simply felt the need to go on a juice fast.

A few minutes into the discussion the man's wife began painting a picture of the physical changes that took place in her husband's body as he detoxified. In three or four days of fasting, his skin began to give off a foul odor and emit a dark ashy substance as the toxins deep within his body were visibly released. His amazing symptoms lasted only for a few days.

He continued sharing his story with Mary. By the end of the month of fasting, he felt better than he had for years. He couldn't remember when he had more energy. He felt truly invigorated, renewed and cleansed—down to the very core of his being.

"That was just six months ago," he said. "But I want to go on another juice fast again just to feel that good again." He was eager to experience the sense of rejuvenation once more.*

YOUR JUICE FASTING PROGRAM

I find it uniquely interesting that this man simply felt the need to go on this fast. Apparently his body was extremely toxic. He may have worked in a toxic environment. Who knows? His inclination to go on an extended juice fast may have spared him from cancer or heart disease several years later. It's impossible to say. But some inner wisdom told him he needed to cleanse his body. I'm glad he listened.

Toxic substances, as we learned earlier, are everywhere. They are in the water that we drink, the air that we breathe and the food that we eat. They attack us from outside and from within.

We are living in the most toxic time the world has ever known. Our ability to stay healthy is increasingly determined by our body's ability to detoxify.

The best way to eliminate these toxins from our bodies is to start a detoxification program. Here's how:

○ Start by following the liver cleansing diet for two to four weeks.

○ Take supplements for a healthy liver.

○ Drink at least two quarts of filtered water.

○ Get plenty of fiber.

○ Undergo periodic juice fasting for two to three days at a time (or longer if monitored by a physician).

○ Finish up with another two weeks on the liver cleansing diet.

---

*This is a dramatized account of a true story.

By following this simple program, you can safely and effectively eliminate the dangerous toxins from your body.

CELLULAR SPRING CLEANING

Periodic fasting is like periodic house cleaning. You may have a regular routine of house cleaning that includes dusting, vacuuming, mopping floors, cleaning bathrooms and a host of other chores. But once or twice a year, many people go after the hidden dirt and grime. They wash curtains, pull furniture away from the walls, wash windows, scrub out cabinets and don't miss a nook or cranny until everything shines.

Our bodies aren't much different. They need regular, thorough cleanings to function at peak efficiency.

The longer we live on this toxic earth, the more we absorb and collect toxins in our tissues. These toxins are actually stored in the tissues of our bodies, especially in the fatty tissues. The liver also stores some toxins that it cannot break down and excrete. Believe it or not, the metabolite of DDT, called DDE, is present in most people's fat.

Fasting is an effective way to help your body eliminate these toxins.

THE WONDERS OF JUICE

The USDA, the Surgeon General, the National Cancer Institute, as well as the U. S. Department of Health and Human Services, all recommend that we eat plenty of fruits and vegetables. In fact, the USDA advises that we eat three to five servings of vegetables plus two to four servings of fruit a day in order to maintain health. This is potentially nine cups of vegetables and fruit a day.[1]

The minimum amount of fruits and vegetables recommended a day is five—three vegetables and two fruits. Less than one-third of Americans get the minimum of five servings a day. Because we eat so little fruit and vegetables, many

Americans suffer from nutritional deficiencies, including vitamin and mineral deficiencies. Common deficiencies include folic acid deficiencies in both men and women. In fact, 60 percent of older Americans do not get enough folic acid to prevent elevated homocysteine levels, which is a risk factor for heart disease.[2]

To make matters worse, the most common vegetables that Americans eat are potatoes in the form of French fries, onions in the form of fried onion rings and tomatoes in the form of ketchup. Even our fresh vegetables are losing their vitamin and mineral content. When we compare the USDA food tables from twenty-five to thirty years ago to the food tables of today, we will see that the nutrient value for over a dozen fruits and vegetables has dropped dramatically.

For example, nearly half the vitamin A and calcium in broccoli have disappeared. In other words, there is about a 50 percent drop in these nutrients in broccoli as compared to the USDA handbook twenty-five to thirty years ago.

VITAL VEGETABLES

Fruits and vegetables are power-packed with phytonutrients, antioxidants, vitamins and minerals that prevent cancer, heart disease, strokes, osteoporosis and most other degenerative diseases.

Do all you can to eat more fruits and vegetables. Since most of us don't have the time to eat the raw fruits and vegetables, it is much simpler to begin juicing fruits and vegetables on a daily basis.

By juicing fresh fruits and vegetables, the juices are separated from the fiber and are quickly digested, absorbed and assimilated by the body. Juice every day to be sure you get plenty of fruits and vegetables. Eight ounces of carrot juice provide the carotenoids that are equal to approximately one and a half pounds of carrots. It would take quite a bit of time to prepare and eat that many carrots every day.

Another excellent way to get adequate amounts of vegetables is through Green Superfood. (See Appendix C.) One scoop is approximately equivalent to six servings of vegetables. I recommend this at least once a day in the morning.

When you get in the daily habit of juicing fruit and vegetables, you can be sure you're getting the recommended three to five servings of vegetables a day and two to four servings of fruit a day that you need. Not only will you learn to love starting your day with delicious fruit and vegetable juices, but you will also dramatically reduce your risk of heart disease, cancer, stroke, diabetes, osteoporosis and macular degeneration.

Give your body the fuel that it craves most—fresh fruits and vegetables—in a form that is easily digested, absorbed and assimilated. You can do this through freshly squeezed juices.

ENZYME ENERGY

Fresh juices are full of enzymes. Enzymes are actually organic compounds or catalysts that increase the rate at which food is broken down and absorbed by the body. Fresh fruits and vegetables are extremely high in enzymes. These enzymes are destroyed during cooking and processing. Bottled and packaged juices are pasteurized, which destroys the enzymes. Fresh juice contains living digestive enzymes that are important in breaking down foods in the digestive tract. This preserves your own body's digestive enzymes. This, in turn, gives your digestive system a much needed rest so that it can repair, recuperate and be rejuvenated.

Eating fats, protein and starch puts a lot of strain on the digestive tract. Recall eating a large T-bone steak and potato with butter or sour cream along with bread and a dessert. Did you get sleepy an hour or two later? That was because that large meal sat in your stomach for hours as the body expended tremendous energy to digest it.

Cooked, starchy foods such as mashed potatoes, breads and pasta contain no enzymes. Therefore, they draw from the enzymes that are produced in the pancreas and deplete your energy.

However, when you drink freshly juiced fruits and vegetables that are teeming with live enzymes, valuable pancreatic enzymes are preserved, giving your pancreas a break.

Juicing pineapples even gives you extra enzyme energy. Pineapples contain the enzyme bromelain, which has been used for decades in treating inflammatory problems such as arthritis, improving wound healing, aiding digestion and numerous other clinical and therapeutic applications.

PHYTO POWER!

But the most important nutrients in fresh fruits and juices are the phytonutrients. Phytonutrients are simply plant-derived nutrients that contain antioxidants. Here are some of the incredible things these mighty plant nutrients can do:

○ Fight tumors and cancer

○ Lower cholesterol

○ Increase immune function

○ Fight viruses

○ Stimulate detoxification enzymes

○ Block the production of cancer-causing compounds

○ Protect the DNA from damage

Many of these phytonutrients are found in the pigments of the fruits and vegetables, such as the chlorophyll of green vegetables, the carotenes or carotenoids in orange fruits and vegetables and the flavonoids in berries.

One out of three Americans will at some time develop

cancer in his or her lifetime. Consuming cruciferous vegetables every day in the form of juices is one of the best ways to protect your body from cancer.

SELECTING YOUR VEGETABLES AND FRUIT FOR JUICING

To prepare your juice for fasting it's important to select the vegetables and fruit that will do you the most good. So let's take a brief look at the major categories of phytonutrients so we can make the healthiest selections.

CAROTENOIDS

First, let's look at the carotenoids. There are more than six hundred. Carotenoids are the fat-soluble pigments you find in red, orange, yellow and dark green fruits and vegetables. Carrots, watermelon, pink grapefruit, sweet potatoes, squash, tomatoes, spinach, kale, collard greens, cantaloupe and yams are bursting with carotenoids. Half of these healthy wonders have the added ability to convert into vitamin A in our livers.

For years, nutritionists taught that the most powerful carotenoid was beta carotene, which is what you find in carrots. Today, we know that other carotenoids have even greater antioxidant and anticancer powers.

The great thing about carotenoids is you can never overdose on them. If you take more than your body needs, the excess will simply not be converted into vitamin A. Instead, it will be stored in your body's fatty tissues and even organs.

Studies have shown that the more carotenoids you take in through your diet, the lower your risk of developing cancer. Wow! That's phyto power![3]

LYCOPENE

Lycopene is a carotenoid found in the red pigment of carrots, tomatoes, pink grapefruit and watermelon. This is a powerful antioxidant that reduces the instance of certain cancers. A study following more than 47,000 individuals found that men who consume large amounts of tomato-based foods each week had significantly lower rates of prostate cancer.[4]

Lycopene is also protective against cancers of the GI tract including the esophagus, stomach, colon and rectum.

LUTEIN

Another very important carotenoid is lutein. This healing substance is found in most yellow fruits and vegetables, such as yellow squash and corn as well as spinach and collard greens.

Lutein protects the eyes from macular degeneration—a major cause of blindness in older individuals.

OTHER CAROTENOIDS

Most of us only know about beta carotene. We feel that we're getting all we need in our daily vitamin pill. But hundreds of other carotenoids exist, including alpha and gamma carotene, Zeaxanthin, canthaxanthin and cryptoxanthin.

We've only begun to scratch the surface in our research about them. But by juicing lots of raw, fresh vegetables, such as carrots, sweet potatoes, collard greens and spinach, we give our bodies a vast array of different carotenoids. Each one of these wholesome vegetables adds another layer of protection from cancer and other degenerative diseases.

CAROTENOIDS AND SMOKING

Even though carotenoids have enormous cancer-fighting properties for nonsmokers, they work just the opposite for smokers.

A large study completed a few years ago showed that supplementation with beta carotene actually increased the instance of lung cancer in smokers. The National Cancer Institute has repeated this study with similar results.[5]

Because of these two startling studies, smokers are warned never to take beta carotene as a supplement. Odd, isn't it? Supplements of beta carotene decrease the incidence of lung cancer in nonsmokers. I believe if the study had used a symphony of antioxidants such as lipoic acid, CoQ_{10}, vitamins E and C, NAC and grape seed extract in addition to the beta carotene, the results would have turned out quite different.

Every time a smoker puffs on a cigarette or cigar he plants a seed for lung cancer. How true the Bible is when it warns that the seeds we sow are the plants we will reap. (See Galatians 6:7.) If you continue to smoke, you will eventually harvest disease—disease that is even fueled by beta carotene.

I once heard a preacher say, "You can still smoke and go to heaven, but you'll just get there a lot sooner!" So, stop smoking and start juicing. Juicing is one of the best ways to break an addiction to cigarettes.

CRUCIFEROUS VEGETABLES

Cruciferous vegetables are cancer blasters. They include cabbage, Brussels sprouts, cauliflower, broccoli, kale, collard greens, mustard greens, turnips and radishes. These cancer fighters contain more phytonutrients with anticancer properties than any other family of vegetables.

The word *cruciferous* comes from the same word root as *crucifying*, which means "to place one on a cross." Oddly, the flowers of cruciferous vegetables contain two components that appear similar to the shape of a cross.

The potent cancer-fighting phytonutrients in the cruciferous vegetables family include indoles, isothiocyanates and sulforaphanes, which are sulfur-containing compounds. They also contain phenols, coumarins, dithiolthiones and glucosinolates, as well as other phytonutrients that are yet to be discovered.

Indoles, especially indole-3-carbinol are potent cancer antagonists. Sulforaphanes stimulate liver detoxification enzymes. Isothiocyanates induce production of detoxification enzymes by the liver, and they prevent damage to the DNA.

Studies have correlated a high intake of cruciferous vegetables, especially cabbage, with lower rates of cancers, especially cancers of the breast and colon.[6]

Broccoli sprouts have the highest concentration of these protective phytonutrients. Select young broccoli sprouts that are about three days old. They contain twenty to fifty times as much of the potent phytonutrient sulforaphane than mature broccoli.

Juicing cruciferous vegetables every day can help your liver to detoxify from pesticides, chemicals, drugs and other pollutants. I encourage you to juice cruciferous vegetables every day of your life—not only during a fast. This is the best insurance policy I know of against cancer.

Even the American Cancer Society recommends eating cruciferous vegetables regularly to decrease your risk of cancer.[7]

FLAVONOIDS

Flavonoids are another group of powerful phytonutrients. They are found in plant pigments, especially blackberries, blueberries, cherries and grapes. More than four thousand different flavonoid compounds give fruits and vegetables their beautiful red, blue and purple color. They are also found in vegetables such as broccoli, tomatoes and peppers.

Isn't it interesting that God placed these beautiful colors in different fruits and vegetables that provide protection from most diseases? Our eyes are actually drawn to the beautiful colors—the brilliant oranges in carrots, the bright reds in tomatoes, the brilliant greens in spinach and other green foods and the brilliant purples and reds in the berries. Really, a big bowl of fresh vegetables is a beautiful sight. Seeing these brilliant flavonoids should entice us to eat them regularly. However, most of us choose dead, processed, manmade foods that are high in sugars, fats and salt and are devoid of these protective phytonutrients.

FLAVONOIDS AND YOUNGER-LOOKING SKIN

Flavonoids can keep your skin looking younger. This is because they play an enormous role in the formation and repair of collagen. Collagen is the major structural protein in the body, and it is also the most abundant protein found in your body. It actually holds the cells and tissues of your body together.

Collagen tends to degenerate with age and slowly collapse, which is why our skin begins to sag as we get older. However, the flavonoids found in berries, cherries, grapes and a host of other fruits and vegetables help to maintain the integrity of your skin's collagen. Therefore, it helps to keep your skin's collagen from degenerating and collapsing with age.

By simply juicing berries and grapes every day, you can get enough flavonoids to nourish your skin's collagen and slow down the aging process.

Flavonoids also help protect you against heart disease.

GRAPE SEED EXTRACT AND PINE BARK EXTRACT

Two flavonoid powerhouses are grape seed extract and pine bark extract. They have twenty times more free-radical scavenger power than vitamin C and fifty times more than vitamin E. The flavonoid phytonutrient in these two extracts is called proanthocyandins. The flavonoid in grape seed extract comes from the seed of the grape, and the flavonoid in pine bark extract comes from the bark of the anneda pine tree.

QUERCETIN

The bioflavonoid quercetin can help your body fight allergies. Allergic conditions include allergic rhinitis, eczema, hives and even some cases of asthma. Quercetin inhibits the release of histamine. Thus, it acts as an antihistamine—but it's all natural! Quercetin is found in onions and apples. No wonder the old saying "An apple a day keeps the doctor away" is true for many since apples are high in quercetin.

Not only are fruits and vegetables full of power-packed flavonoids, many vegetables also contain chlorophyll. Let's look.

CHLOROPHYLL

Chlorophyll comes from the green pigment in plants. Just as the life of a person is in the blood, so the life of a plant is in the chlorophyll. In other words, chlorophyll is like the plant's blood.

Chlorophyll is very high in magnesium. It's vitally important for photosynthesis, which is the way plants convert light into energy. Foods that are high in chlorophyll include greens such as beet greens, spinach, collard greens, parsley and other deep green vegetables. Wheat grass, barley grass, alfalfa, spirulina, chlorella and blue-green algae are plant "superfoods." They are superfoods because of their high chlorophyll content.

These superfoods are also high in flavonoids, which gives them anti-inflammatory, antitumor and antiviral effects. Various algae, including chlorella, spirulina and blue-green algae are very high in carotenoids. In fact, spirulina has about ten times the concentration of carotenoids as carrots. These different algae also contain nearly all the essential amino acids along with practically every mineral and trace mineral that your body needs! Green Superfood contains all of these high-chlorophyll foods. (See Appendix C.)

CHLOROPHYLLIN

Greens such as spinach, collard greens, beet greens and parsley, together with the superfoods, are very high in chlorophyllin. Chlorophyllins fight cancer by inhibiting many different carcinogens. Chlorophyllin can help reduce the cancer-causing substances, called carcinogens, in cooked meats and fried foods. They even help to reduce the carcinogens in cigarette smoke. They also help to protect DNA from radiation damage.

Not only are green foods packed with this vital substance, but also the magnesium levels they contain give them a double punch. Magnesium helps to cleanse the GI tract. As a matter of fact, it works similarly to a mild laxative. Therefore, green foods help your body remove toxins from your GI tract so they are not reabsorbed.

High-chlorophyll foods are effective antioxidants, cancer and tumor fighters, as well as virus fighters. Green food preparations, such as Green Superfood can be added to your freshly squeezed morning juices. (See Appendix C.)

GREEN SUPERFOOD

One scoop of Green Superfood is equal to about six servings of vegetables. Green Superfood contains wheat grass, barley grass, alfalfa, spirulina, chlorella, blue-green algae, along with green tea, grape seed extract, milk thistle and good bacteria. You can give your detox program a turbo charge boost by using this or a similar product during the detox program, during a fast and on a daily basis thereafter.

ALLIUM

Other important phytonutrients are the allium compounds. Garlic contains the highest concentration of these phytonutrients. Allicin is the main allium compound and is what gives garlic its strong odor. Garlic actually has over a hundred different compounds, and they are probably the reason garlic has so many therapeutic effects.

For instance, garlic helps to promote Phase Two detoxification of the liver. It protects against cancer. It has antibacterial, antifungal, antiviral and antiparasitic properties as well. It also helps to detoxify the body of heavy metals such as lead and mercury, and it strengthens the immune system.

Cooking and processing garlic robs it of many of these incredible disease-fighting properties. That's why I recommend juicing garlic to get all its health benefits.

ELLAGIC ACID

Ellagic acid is found in strawberries, raspberries, grapes and black currants. This powerful healing substance has been shown to inhibit cancer that has been chemically induced in rats.[8]

Ellagic acid also blocks against the cancer-causing effects of many different toxins, including compounds in cigarette smoke called PAH. It also protects against damage by toxins to chromosomes, which are our genetic blueprint. Finally, ellagic acid is a powerful antioxidant and can actually increase glutathione levels.

A new method of determining a food's antioxidant capacity is call ORAC (oxygen radical absorbency capacity). Foods with the highest ORAC scores have the greatest ability to neutralize free radicals. Fruits are at the top of the list. The top five foods on the list are prunes, raisins, blueberries, blackberries and garlic. Strawberries are number eight. Broccoli is number fifteen, and tomatoes are number forty-two. Isn't that amazing that blueberries, blackberries and strawberries have a higher antioxidant capacity than most all other fruits and vegetables? (If you eat raisins, make sure they are organic since raisins are usually high in pesticides.)

VITAMINS AND MINERALS THROUGH JUICING

Even though the majority of Americans appear to be healthy, most are not. The majority of Americans are actually taking inadequate amounts of vitamins and minerals.

MAGNESIUM

For example, Americans commonly don't get enough magnesium in their diets. The government says each one of us should get 300–350 milligrams of magnesium a day, but few of us do. Vegetables, especially green leafy vegetables, are very high in magnesium. By juicing green vegetables every day, or by taking Green Superfood, you will be sure to get all the magnesium you need.

Mineral deficiencies are even more common in the standard American diet than vitamin deficiencies. It's also common for women to get too little iron and calcium in their diets.

FOLIC ACID

The most common nutritional deficiency in the world is folic acid deficiency. One reason for this is that we simply don't eat enough vegetables. In addition, some medications, such as birth control pills, contribute to this deficiency. Alcohol and stress can play a part also. Nevertheless, adequate folic acid is vital to good health; without it we stand to increase our risk of heart disease by having elevated levels of homocysteine (a toxic amino acid).

Folic acid is necessary for DNA repair, and it keeps your immune system strong. Studies have shown that high doses of folic acid can eliminate most of the precancerous cells on women with cervical dysplasia.[9] Dark green leafy vegetables, such as spinach and collard greens, are excellent sources of folic acid.

VITAMIN C

Even though severe vitamin C deficiency and scurvy are extremely rare in the United States and other countries, marginal deficiencies are relatively common. I believe this plays a role in the development of diseases such as heart disease and cancer. Excellent sources of vitamin C include freshly juiced citrus fruit such as grapefruit and oranges. Other sources include kiwi, strawberries, broccoli and Brussels sprouts.

Vitamin C is easily lost during both cooking and storage of the food. Vitamin C from natural sources contains bioflavonoids, which enhance the effect of vitamin C.

Juicing a wide variety of fruits and vegetables will assure you of getting enough of most all vitamins and minerals.

COMING ATTRACTIONS

These are just a few of the recent nutritional breakthrough discoveries found by researchers. Nutritional medicine is still in its infancy, but what we've learned thus far is truly exciting.

Without a doubt, many more important phytonutrients will be discovered and will offer more protection against cancer, heart disease and other degenerative diseases.

But don't wait for scientific proof—start juicing today. Nevertheless, I want to encourage you to begin using these powerful phytonutrients every day by daily juicing fresh fruits and vegetables. They will play a major role in your detox fast, but don't stop there. Determine that after your fast is over you will make juicing fresh fruits and vegetables a part of your daily breakfast routine.

The research that we have already should convince each of us of the overwhelming healing power and health benefits of fresh, raw fruits and vegetables. Don't wait for more studies. Start making use of this life-saving wisdom right now!

SIX

Dr. C's
Detox Fast

You stagger into the kitchen half asleep, dragging the belt of your robe behind you like a long tail. Too groggy to speak, you pull your juicer out from a lower cabinet, plunk it on the counter and reach for the apples, carrots and other fruits and vegetables piled high in a giant bowl.

With the water running, you clean and chop the colorful ingredients of your first day's juice fast menu. In minutes, your juicer is whirring, spinning and extracting the elements of your brand-new, healthier, detoxified lifestyle.

It's done. You slowly, carefully touch your lips to the glass, wondering if you'll be able to drink this concoction you just made. But as you touch it to your tongue, you're amazed. It's more than delicious—it's delightful and refreshing. You had been willing to grit your teeth and endure this juicing program because you were convinced of its benefits to your health. But you never dreamed you'd enjoy it so much!

I genuinely believe that you are going to find this fasting program more enjoyable, easier and more rewarding than you ever expected. Not only that, but when you are through, your renewed energy and vitality will amaze you.

So let's get started with the juice fast portion of this detoxification program.

BEFORE YOUR FAST

Before beginning the actual juice fasting portion of this program, you should have been following the diet to support your liver for about two weeks (four weeks for those with extreme toxicity). As you've seen already, you will want to go back on the liver support diet for the same period of time following your juice fast.

If you've completed the liver support diet, you're ready to detox. So, let's get started. Here are some pointers:

○ As you begin, you should already have increased your intake of filtered water to two quarts a day. Continue drinking at least two quarts per day of filtered water throughout the duration of your fast.

○ During the fast, I do not recommend consuming vitamins. You should have taken a number of vitamins and minerals during your two-week-long liver support diet. You must stop taking all of these supplements until your fasting period is over. Afterward, you will go back on the liver support diet for two additional weeks. At that point, you will need to resume taking these supplements until the two-week period is ended. You should continue taking a comprehensive multivitamin, a comprehensive antioxidant and a chlorophyll drink daily even after completing the program.

HOW LONG SHOULD I FAST?

Periodic, short fasts of two to three days are an excellent way to detoxify your body. And using the guidelines provided, they are extremely safe. Fasting for longer than three days should only be done under a doctor's supervision.

I usually recommend that patients start out by fasting one day and gradually work up to three days. However, under a doctor's supervision, this fast can be continued for one to two weeks or even longer.

Detox fasting should be done several times a year. Once again—repeated fasts for three days are usually enough time to cleanse the body.

WATCH OUT FOR . . .

Fasting can produce some interesting changes in your body, so be aware of this before you begin. Some of these changes are more common than others. So, here are some precautions you need to consider.

○ *You may experience lightheadedness.* Lightheadedness is common. Therefore, don't rise up suddenly from lying or sitting during your fast period. You may even experience some dizziness if you stand up too quickly. If you do get lightheaded, lie down and elevate your feet on a few pillows.

○ *You may experience changes in energy.* Some people become very fatigued during a fast. Others feel much more energetic. Don't be alarmed if you experience either of these extremes. Initially you may be fatigued, but energy levels increase as you detox.

○ *Your sleep habits may change.* You may not need as much sleep at night as normal. Don't be alarmed.

○ *You should get plenty of rest.* During a fast, you will need plenty of rest, both during the day and at night. Be prepared to take a siesta in the afternoon for about an hour to an hour and a half, if possible. Some people may even need a morning nap.

○ *You should limit activity.* I do not recommend any strenuous exercise during the fast. Take strolls in a park, walk on a beach or enjoy any other slow, relaxing activities.

○ *Constipation can be a problem.* Constipation is also common, especially during longer fasts. (You probably won't experience constipation on short, juice fasts.) For this I recommend juicing pitted prunes or pitted plums along with apples. Or you may drink herbal teas, which we will discuss in the next section. Also, mixing one scoop of Green Superfood in one of the juices helps prevent constipation.

If you still cannot have a bowel movement, I strongly recommend using an enema. For severely constipated patients I recommend at least one enema a day. Simply fill an enema bag with luke-warm water. One pint to one quart of water is usually enough. Then follow the instructions on the enema box. It is best to first lie on your back for a minute or so, then on your right side, then on the stomach, and then finally on your left side. Gently massage your stomach at the same time. If you still have problems with constipa-tion, I recommend that you see a colon therapist who is able to administer colonics or colenemas.

○ *You may have cold hands and feet.* During a fast it's common to experience a lowering of body temperature, which may make your hands and feet feel cold. Don't be concerned. Simply use an extra blanket at night and wear extra clothing.

○ *Your tongue may become coated.* Another very common symptom during fasting is coating of the tongue. Your tongue may develop a white or yellow film. This film signals you that your body is detoxifying.

○ *You may experience bad breath.* Your breath may take on an unpleasant odor as your body detoxifies. Just keep a toothbrush with you, and brush your teeth and tongue often with organic toothpaste such as Tom's of Maine brand.

○ *Skin eruptions may occur.* Acne, boils and rashes are other signs that your body is excreting toxins through your skin, which is the body's largest excretory organ.

○ *Body odor may be a problem.* Some people even develop an offensive body odor as poisons exit the body through the sweat glands.

○ *Nausea and vomiting may also occur during a fast.* This is usually a sign that you've become mildly dehydrated. That's why getting enough fluids is critically important during your fast.

○ *Your urine may appear darker than normal.* This also usually means that your body is shedding poisons or that you are not consuming adequate liquids. So if this occurs, increase your fluid intake.

○ *You may have added mucous drainage from your sinuses, bronchial tubes and even the GI tract.* Don't be alarmed by this. Once again, these symptoms are usually just your body's way of voiding itself of many of the built-up toxins it has been storing.

LET'S GET STARTED

To get started on your fast, you will want to purchase lots of fresh, organically grown vegetables and fruits. I have provided a shopping list of vegetables for you to take to the store at the end this chapter.

Organic vegetables are the best because they are grown without pesticides and herbicides. Since you are fasting to remove such chemicals, it's important not to take any in during your fast. I believe organic produce is the safest. It can be found at many of the larger health food stores. There are even health food stores that are as large as some supermarkets such as Whole Foods and Wild Oats. These have a wide variety of organic fruits and vegetables at a competitive price.

In addition, many of the larger supermarkets are beginning to stock organic produce as the public is demanding it. Our voices will be heard if we continue to ask the supermarket to carry organic products.

WHAT IF I CAN'T USE ORGANICS?

Nevertheless, organic vegetables tend to be more expensive, and they can be difficult to find. If you can't always use organics, then you must take special care to clean your fruits and vegetables to remove all waxes and chemicals.

Growers are free to use about four hundred different pesticides on crops. Each year in the United States, over one billion pounds of pesticides and herbicides are sprayed on the food we eat. Pesticides that have been banned in the United States are often shipped to other Third World countries. Fruits and vegetables grown in these countries are sprayed with pesticides banned in the United States and then exported from those countries back into the United States.

So here are some rules to remember when purchasing fruits and vegetables.

LOOK FOR THICKER PEELS

Usually, the thicker the peel, the safer the fruit. For example, bananas have thick peels and generally have little pesticide in the actual fruit. That is, unless they are grown in Third World countries where more potent pesticides can be used, which can penetrate the entire fruit.

Oranges, tangerines, lemons, grapefruits and watermelons are also excellent fruits since they have a thicker peel.

PRODUCE WITH THIN PEELS

Fruits and vegetables with thin peels or none at all usually contain higher pesticide residue. These include apples, grapes, peaches, strawberries, kiwi, cherries, blackberries, blueberries, broccoli, lettuce, carrots and corn. Fruits and vegetables with some of the highest levels of pesticides include tomatoes, spinach and potatoes.

In addition to the pesticides that are sprayed on the plants, waxes are added to keep the produce from spoiling. Unfortunately for us, most of these waxes contain pesticides and fungicides, too. These seal water in and prevent the produce from spoiling.

WASHING OFF PRODUCE WAXES

If you've ever tried, I'm sure you found that these waxes are pretty difficult to remove. In fact, they usually can't be removed by simply washing them with water.

SPECIALLY PREPARED CLEANSERS

You can purchase a natural, biodegradable cleanser from most health food stores. Use it to gently scrub off the wax, and then rinse the produce off. You may also simply soak your produce in a mild detergent such as Ivory or pure castille soap from a health food store. Gently scrub your fruits and vegetables and rinse them off.

Hydrogen peroxide

Another way to remove pesticides is to soak the fruits and vegetables in a sink of cold water. Then add one tablespoon of 35 percent, food-grade hydrogen peroxide (which can be purchased at a health food store) to the water. The sink should be approximately half-filled. Allow the produce to soak for five to fifteen minutes. Then rinse them thoroughly with fresh water.

Soak fruits with thin peels and leafy vegetables for only five minutes or so. Thicker vegetables, such as carrots and other fibrous vegetables, should be soaked for ten to fifteen minutes.

Clorox bleach

Believe it or not, another good way to remove pesticides is to soak your produce in a sink half full of cold water. Then add one teaspoon of Clorox bleach. It must be the Clorox regular bleach, not a generic brand. Soak them for the same amount of time as above, and rinse them thoroughly for about three to five minutes.

CHOOSE A JUICER

You may start with an inexpensive juicer such as a Juice Man juicer from Wal-Mart, which costs about $70. There are many different types of juicers, and some are very expensive. The Champion juicer is an excellent juicer and will usually last for decades. The Vita-Mix is a different type of juicer that looks more like a large blender. (See Appendix C.) It is able to completely juice and liquify the entire fruit or vegetable. This has the added benefit of providing the fiber in addition to the vitamins, minerals, antioxdants, enzymes and phytonutrients. However, it is more expensive, usually costing over $400. I personally have all three types of juicers.

GUIDELINES FOR YOUR FAST

THE DAY BEFORE YOUR FAST

On the day before your juice fast, prepare yourself for the fast by eating only fruits and vegetables.

FAST ON THE WEEKENDS

I strongly recommend that you begin your juice fast on the weekend. By doing so, you will be able to spend more time resting. If you experience any side effects such as fatigue, lightheadedness or a headache, it will not interfere with your job (since it is the weekend).

The more you are able to rest during a fast, the better. I commonly tell patients who are sick to rest since, if they continue to work or exercise, the energy that would be used for healing is diverted for other body activities. Therefore, during the fast it is best to rest so that your energy can be directed at healing and detoxifying.

DON'T USE PREPARED JUICES

It's very important that you juice raw, fresh fruits and vegetables. Don't try to do this fast by purchasing prepared juices. They are simply not the same. Fresh juice contains the living enzymes, phytonutrients, antioxidants, vitamins and minerals. Bottled, canned and processed juices have been pasteurized. Many of the phytonutrients and enzymes have been lost in the process.

DON'T DRINK ALCOHOL, COFFEE OR SOFT DRINKS

During your fast, drink only juices and herbal teas. You may also sip soup broth by gently warming vegetable juice. Limit teas to herbal teas and green tea. Also, drink plenty of filtered water, about two quarts a day.

SIP JUICES SLOWLY

When drinking your specially prepared juices, sip them slowly to mix the juice with saliva. Don't gulp them down.

PREPARING PRODUCE

Peel oranges and grapefruits, but be sure and leave on the white, pithy part of the peel. That is the part that contains the important bioflavonoids.

Leave the skins on all other fruits and vegetables. Remove the green top portion from carrots, since they may contain a toxic substance. Slice the fruits and vegetables so that they fit nicely into your juicer.

Drink the juices immediately after juicing—do not store them. As soon as a fruit or vegetable is sliced, it begins to lose nutritional value. For instance, cut an apple and place it on a dish on your counter. You will notice that it doesn't take long to turn brown. This is due to oxidation from exposure to the air.

When you slice cucumbers, they lose about 40 to 50 percent of their vitamin C content within the first few hours. A cantaloupe that has been sliced will lose about a third of its vitamin C content within a day. That's why it is always best to drink fruit and vegetable juices immediately to get the maximum nutritional benefits. Do not try to store them.

BEST FRUIT AND VEGGIE CHOICES

When you're juicing, keep in mind that some fruits and vegetables provide more health benefits than others.

Fruits and veggies that are especially cleansing on the juice fast include:

Ŏ Cabbage and other cruciferous vegetables

Ŏ Greens

Ŏ Dandelion root and dandelion greens

Ŏ Sprouts

Ŏ Celery

Ŏ Carrots

○ Lemons and limes

○ Apples

○ Beets

○ Berries (blueberries, blackberries and strawberries). Caution: Some people may be allergic to berries.

For optimum detoxification, drink one juice drink a day that contains cruciferous vegetables such as cabbage or broccoli and beets. The phytonutrients in these vegetables help detoxify your body by helping to detox your liver and enhancing the flow of bile. Include dandelion greens or dandelion root to support your liver in its detoxification efforts during the fast, too.

THE BASICS OF JUICE FASTING

IN THE MORNING AND FOR LUNCH
Juice fruits and vegetables.

IN THE AFTERNOON AND EVENING
Juice veggies.

In the next few pages you will find numerous delicious and healthful juicing combinations. However, they are simply guides to help you find your own favorites. Be creative! Make your own combinations and experiment with juicing.

When you create your own juices, there are four main fruits and vegetables that should usually form the base of each juice. These include:

○ Carrots

○ Celery

○ Apples

○ Tomatoes

One of these, or a combination of them, should make up

the greatest portion of your juice. You will find that they taste good and combine well with other fruits and vegetables. In addition, they are able to disguise the taste of veggies you may not like, such as cabbage and greens.

When you add greens, such as collard greens, spinach, broccoli, parsley, wheat grass or dandelion greens, they should make up no more than one quarter of the juice. If you use more, you may not enjoy the taste. The recipes should make 8–12 ounces of juice, but some may make 16 ounces, depending on the size of your fruits and vegetables.

SUGGESTED JUICING RECIPES

BREAKFAST JUICES

BREAKFAST DRINK 1
½ small lemon or lime, peeled
1 cup berries
3 oranges, peeled
1 scoop Green Superfood (optional)

BREAKFAST DRINK 2
4 carrots
A handful of parsley
2 apples
1 scoop Green Superfood (optional)

BREAKFAST DRINK 3
1 pink grapefruit, peeled
½ small lemon or lime, peeled
1 apple
1 scoop Green Superfood (optional)

BREAKFAST DRINK 4
4 carrots
1 apple
1 beet
1 scoop Green Superfood (optional)

Breakfast Drink 5
2 apples
¼-inch slice ginger root
½ small lemon or lime
1 scoop Green Superfood (optional)
Add water to equal 8 oz.

Breakfast Drink 6
1 cup strawberries, blueberries or blackberries
1 pink grapefruit, peeled
1 scoop Green Superfood (optional)

MIDMORNING JUICE SNACKS

Snack Drink 1
2 celery stalks
2 apples
2 carrots

Snack Drink 2
A handful of parsley
4 carrots
1 apple

Snack Drink 3
2 carrots
2 celery stalks
1 apple
1 beet

Snack Drink 4
3-inch slice pineapple with skin
¼-inch ginger root
A handful of parsley

Snack Drink 5
4 carrots
A handful of spinach, collard greens or beet greens
1 apple

SNACK DRINK 6
Cut watermelon in sections.
Juice enough watermelon to equal 8–12 oz. of juice.

SNACK DRINK 7
½ cantaloupe
1 cup berries

LUNCH JUICES

LUNCH JUICE 1
2 celery stalks
4 carrots
A handful of parsley
1 garlic clove

LUNCH JUICE 2
1 beet
2 carrots
2 celery stalks
½ sweet potato (uncooked)

LUNCH JUICE 3
¼–½ head of cabbage
A handful of collard greens
2 carrots
1 apple

LUNCH JUICE 4
A handful of parsley
1 tomato
1 cucumber
2 celery stalks
1 garlic clove (optional)

LUNCH JUICE 5
1 handful of dandelion greens or 1 dandelion root
2 celery stalks
4 carrots

LUNCH JUICE 6
2 celery stalks
2 carrots
1 beet
¼–½ cabbage

EVENING JUICES

EVENING JUICE 1
¼–½ cabbage
2 stalks celery
½ cucumber

EVENING JUICE 2
4 medium tomatoes
2 celery stalks
½ cucumber
1 handful of alfalfa sprouts or broccoli sprouts
1 garlic clove (optional)

EVENING JUICE 3
2 carrots
1 beet
½ cucumber
2 celery stalks

EVENING JUICE 4
4 carrots
A handful of collard greens, spinach or beet greens
1 garlic clove
A handful of parsley

EVENING JUICE 5
4 carrots
A handful of dandelion greens or 1 dandelion root

CRUCIFEROUS VEGGIES ARE IMPORTANT!

I want to emphasize that it is critically important to drink at least one juice drink with cabbage or broccoli and one juice drink with beets each day to increase and support liver detoxification as well as to enhance the flow of bile.

Any of the vegetable combinations can also be juiced first and then slowly warmed. Don't overheat them. Then you may have them as soup. However, never boil the juices, for that will destroy their enzymes. Take them off the stove before they boil. They should be warm, not hot. If you have a Vita-Mix juicer, the juicer has the ability to heat up the juice through rapid spinning.

SOUPS

Soup 1

2 garlic cloves
½ cucumber
2 celery stalks
A handful of spinach

Soup 2

4 carrots
2 celery stalks
A handful of parsley
1 garlic clove

Soup 3

2 tomatoes
1 cucumber
2 celery stalks
1 garlic clove

Soup 4

¼–½ head of cabbage
2 celery stalks
2 carrots
A handful of parsley

SOUP 5

1 cucumber
2 tomatoes
A handful of parsley
1 garlic clove

TO SPICE IT UP

You may add a dash of Tabasco sauce and/or dulse powder. Dulse is a very tasty, salty seaweed that has a red/purple leaf. It is high in potassium, calcium, iron and iodine, and it is used in soups and salads.

HERB TEAS

MILK THISTLE TEA AND DANDELION TEA

Certain herbs are very important for supporting the liver in detoxification during the fast. Other herbs are important for supporting the kidneys and the GI tract. Milk thistle and dandelion tea are very important in supporting the liver for detoxification.

Milk thistle actually protects the liver from toxins, and dandelion helps to increase bile production and stimulate the gallbladder to excrete the bile. Drink milk thistle tea every day during your fast along with dandelion tea to protect the liver and to help rid the body of bile, which contains many of the toxins.

Herb teas can be sweetened with a small amount of Stevia, which can be found in most health food stores.

ASPARAGUS TEA AND NETTLE TEA

Since toxins are eliminated primarily through the kidneys and GI tract, it is critically important to support the kidneys during a fast. Asparagus tea along with nettle tea has diuretic properties. This also helps to support the kidneys so that they can eliminate toxins more effectively.

GREEN TEA

Green tea is very high in polyphenols called catechins. This tea has 200 times more antioxidant power than vitamin E and 500 times more than vitamin C. Green tea does contain caffeine, however. So, don't drink it too late in the day or it can interfere with sleep. I strongly recommend that you enjoy green tea in the morning and for lunch.

CHAMOMILE TEA

Chamomile tea benefits digestion and also has calming properties. It is an excellent tea to drink after dinner to help calm you before going to bed.

SLEEPY TIME TEA

Sleepy Time tea is an effective herbal remedy for those who suffer from insomnia.

SMOOTH MOVE TEA

Smooth Move tea is an excellent herbal tea to temporarily help with regularity during a juice fast.

BREAKING YOUR FAST

Breaking your fast often is the most difficult and most important part of fasting. Therefore, you must understand how to break your fast before you even begin.

You must reintroduce foods gradually to realize the greatest health benefits of fasting. You see, your digestive tract has been at rest. That means hydrochloric acid and pancreatic enzymes may not be available to help you digest proteins, starches and fats right away. Therefore, the longer your fast time, the more slowly you should come off of your fast.

Here's an eating schedule for coming off of your fast if your fast is three days or longer. If the fast is only one or two days, you can eat fruit the first day, then go on the liver support diet for two weeks as outlined in chapter 8.

THE FIRST DAY AFTER YOUR FAST

Eat fresh fruit such as apples, watermelon, grapes or fresh berries as often as every two to three hours on the first day that your fast is broken.

However, don't eat papaya or pineapple on the first day after a fast. These fruits contain strong enzymes that may upset your stomach. Fruits with the highest water content, such as watermelon, are the easiest to digest.

THE SECOND DAY AFTER YOUR FAST

On the second day after the fast is broken, have fruit in the morning. For lunch and dinner, have a bowl of fresh vegetable soup for lunch and for dinner.

Eat slowly and chew your food very well. Be sure not to overeat.

Be sure you continue to drink at least two quarts of filtered water a day. You may also continue to drink your juices once or twice a day.

DAY THREE AFTER YOUR FAST

On the third day, you may add to the fruit and vegetable soup a salad and/or a baked potato. You may also add a slice of whole-grain bread such as Ezekiel bread, brown rice bread or millet bread.

DAY FOUR AFTER YOUR FAST

On the fourth day, you may introduce a small amount (1 or 2 ounces) of free-range chicken, turkey, fish or free-range lean meat.

Just remember, the key is eating slowly and chewing very well. Drink water thirty minutes before your meal, but not more than 4 ounces with your meal. Most importantly– don't overeat.

SPECIAL ADVICE FOR SPECIAL PROBLEMS

Not everyone who begins a fasting program is in the same

healthy state. You may have some physical problems that you need to address before beginning to fast. Therefore, be on the lookout for these special problems before starting this fasting program.

CANDIDIASIS, FOOD ALLERGIES, PARASITES

If you regularly experience excessive bloating, gas and diarrhea, you may be suffering from candidiasis, bacterial overgrowth in the small intestines or even a parasitic infection. You may also be suffering from malabsorption, maldigestion, increased intestinal permeability, food allergies or food sensitivities.

If you have any of these symptoms, I strongly recommend getting a comprehensive digestive stool analysis with parasitology, a test for intestinal permeability and a food allergy test. (See Appendix C.)

In addition, I recommend that you read my booklet *The Bible Cure for Candida and Yeast Infections* and follow the special diet it contains for three months before you start fasting.

HYPOGLYCEMIA

If you have hypoglycemia, grind 1 tablespoon of flaxseeds, or take another form of fiber, and add it to your juice. Juice every two to three hours instead of juicing only four or five times a day.

You can place 1 tablespoon of flaxseeds into a coffee grinder and grind them. Other good sources of fiber include rice bran, psyllium seeds or husks and oat bran.

SENSITIVE GI TRACT

I have found that patients with very sensitive GI tracts do better when they separate fruit juices from vegetable juice.

If you experience pain, bloating, gas or diarrhea after drinking one of the juices, simply omit that juice and try a different one. By process of elimination, you can find what fruit or vegetable is causing the problem. When you identify the item to which you are sensitive, simply eliminate it from your juice fast.

SELECTING FRUITS AND VEGETABLES ACCORDING TO YOUR BLOOD TYPE

Another solution for individuals with sensitive GI tracts is to eat fruits and vegetables according to your blood type. You can find out your blood type by donating blood at the local blood bank or by going to your doctor.

For each individual blood type there are fruits and vegetables that are very beneficial, some that are neutral and fruits and vegetables that one should avoid.[1]

Here's a list of blood-type fruits and vegetables to get you started.

TYPE A

HIGHLY BENEFICIAL

Vegetables: Artichokes, beet leaves, broccoli, carrots, chicory, collard greens, dandelion, escarole, garlic, horseradish, kale, kohlrabi, leek, lettuce, romaine, okra, onions (red, Spanish, yellow), parsley, parsnips, pumpkin, spinach, sprouts (alfalfa), Swiss chard, tempeh, tofu, turnips.

Fruits: Apricots, blackberries, blueberries, cherries, cranberries, figs, grapefruit, lemons, pineapple, plums, prunes, raisins.

NEUTRAL

Vegetables: Arugula, asparagus, avocado, bamboo shoots, beets, bok choy, caraway, cauliflower, celery, chervil, coriander, corn, cucumber, daikon radish, dill, endive, fennel, fiddlehead ferns, ginger, lettuces, mushrooms (enoki, portobello, oyster), mustard greens, olives (green), onions (green), radicchio, radishes, rappini, rutabaga, scallions/shallots, seaweed, sprouts (Brussels, mung, radish), squash (all types), water chestnut, watercress, zucchini.

Fruits: Apples, currants, dates, elderberries, grapes (all kinds), guava, kiwi, kumquat, limes, loganberries, melon (canang, casaba, Christmas, Crenshaw, musk, Spanish, watermelon), nectarine, peaches, pears, persimmons, pomegranates, prickly pear, starfruit, strawberries.

AVOID

Vegetables: Cabbage (Chinese, red, white), eggplant, lima beans, mushrooms (domestic, shiitake), mustard greens, olives (black, Greek, Spanish), peppers (green, jalapeno, red, yellow), potatoes (sweet, red, white), tomatoes, yams.

Fruits: Bananas, coconuts, mangoes, melon (cantaloupe, honeydew), oranges, papayas, plantains, rhubarb, tangerines.[2]

TYPE B

HIGHLY BENEFICIAL

Vegetables: Beets, beet leaves, broccoli, cabbage (Chinese, red, white), carrots, cauliflower, collard greens, eggplant, kale, lima beans, mushrooms (shiitake), mustard greens, parsley, parsnips, peppers (green, red, jalapeno, red, yellow), potatoes (sweet), sprouts (Brussels), yams.

Fruits: Bananas, cranberries, grapes (black, concord, green, red), papaya, pineapple, plums.

NEUTRAL

Vegetables: Arugula, asparagus, avocado, bamboo shoots, bok choy, celery, chervil, chicory, cucumber, daikon radish, dandelion, dill, endive, escarole, fennel, fiddlehead ferns, garlic, ginger, horseradish, kohlrabi, leek, lettuce (all types), mushrooms (domestic, enoki, portobello, tree oyster), okra, onions (green, red, Spanish, yellow), radicchio, rappini, rutabaga, scallions, seaweed, shallots, snow peas, spinach, sprouts (alfafa), Swiss chard, turnips, water chestnuts, watercress, zucchini.

Fruits: Apples, apricots, blackberries, blueberries, boysenberries, cherries, currants, dates, elderberries, figs, gooseberries, grapefruit, guava, kiwi, kumquat, lemons, limes, loganberries, melon (all types), nectarines, oranges, peaches, raisins, pears, prunes, plantains, strawberries, tangerines.

Avoid

Vegetables: Artichokes (domestic and Jerusalem), avocado, corn (yellow, white), olives (black, green, Greek, Spanish), pumpkin, radishes, sprouts (mung, radish), tempeh, tofu, tomato.

Fruits: Coconuts, persimmons, pomegranates, prickly pear, rhubarb, starfruit.[3]

TYPE AB

Highly beneficial

Vegetables: Beet leaves, beets, broccoli, cauliflower, celery, collard greens, cucumber, dandelion, garlic, kale, mustard greens, eggplant, parsley, parsnips, potatoes (sweet), sprouts (alfalfa), tempeh, tofu, yams.

Fruits: Cherries, cranberries, figs, grapes, kiwi, loganberries, gooseberries, grapefruit, lemons, pineapple, plums, prunes.

Neutral

Vegetables: Arugula, asparagus, bamboo shoots, horseradish, bok choy, cabbage (red, Chinese, white), caraway, carrots, chervil, coriander, daikon radish, dill, endive, escarole, fennel, fiddlehead ferns, tomato, ginger, lettuce, leeks, mushrooms, potatoes (red, white), okra, pumpkin, olives (green, Spanish), onions (all), radicchio, rappini, rutabaga, shallots, scallions, snow peas, seaweed, sprouts (Brussels, mung, radish), squash (all types), water chestnut, watercress, zucchini.

Fruits: Apples, apricots, berries (black, blue), boysenberries, currants, dates, elderberries, kumquats, limes, papayas, tangerines, melon (cantaloupe, casaba, Christmas, crenshaw, musk, Spanish, watermelons), nectarine, peaches, pears, plantains, prunes, raisins, raspberries, strawberries.

Avoid

Vegetables: Artichokes, corn, avocado, lima beans, mushrooms (shiitake), olives (black), peppers (green, jalapeno, red, yellow), sprouts (mung, radish).

97

Fruits: Bananas, coconuts, guava, mangoes, oranges, persimmons, pomegranates, prickly pears, rhubarb, starfruit.[4]

TYPE O

HIGHLY BENEFICIAL

Vegetables: Artichokes, beet leaves, broccoli, chicory, collard greens, dandelion, escarole, garlic, horseradish, kale, kohlrabi, leek, lettuce (romaine), okra, onions (red, Spanish, yellow), parsley, parsnips, peppers (red), potatoes (sweet), pumpkin, seaweed, spinach, Swiss chard, turnips.

Fruits: Figs, plums, prunes.

NEUTRAL

Vegetables: Arugula, asparagus, bamboo shoots, beet, bok choy, caraway, celery, carrots, chervil, coriander, cucumber, daikin, dill, endive, fennel, fiddlehead ferns, ginger, lettuce, lima beans, mushrooms (enoki, portobello, oyster), olives (green), onions (green), peppers (green, yellow, jalapeno), radicchio, radishes, rappini, rutabaga, scallions, shallots, snow peas, sprouts (mung, radish), squash (all types), tempeh, tofu, tomato, water chestnut, watercress, yams, zucchini.

Fruits: Apples, apricots, bananas, blueberries, boysenberries, cherries, cranberries, currants, dates, elderberries, gooseberries, grapefruit, grapes, guava, kiwi, kumquat, lemons, limes, mangoes, melons (casaba, Crenshaw, musk, watermelon), nectarines, papayas, peaches, pears, persimmons, pineapples, pomegranates, prickly pear, raisins, raspberries, starfruit.

AVOID

Vegetables: Avocado, cabbage (Chinese, red, white), cauliflower, corn (white, yellow), eggplant, mushroom (domestic, shiitake), mustard greens, olives (black, Greek, Spanish), potatoes (red, white), sprouts (alfalfa, Brussels).

Fruits: Blackberries, coconuts, melon (cantaloupe, honeydew), oranges, plantains, rhubarb, strawberries, tangerines.[5]

98

I encourage you to experiment with the many wonderful, delicious and healthy fruits and vegetables offered above. Don't just stop when your fast period ends; consider making juicing an ongoing lifestyle. For more recipes I also recommend the book by Jay Kordich, *The Juiceman's Power of Juicing*. However, be sure to juice cabbage or broccoli, beets, and other of the potent detoxifying and antioxidant fruits and veggies daily in order to help the body detoxify, cleanse and heal.

CONSIDER MAKING JUICING A LIFESTYLE

Many believe that they can fast one time and go back to eating the same high-fat, high-sugar, high-processed starches and high-meat diet that caused them to develop the degenerative diseases in the first place. That would be the same as saying that if a person stopped smoking for a month, then he could go back and start smoking his two packs of cigarettes a day. Don't go back to the old unhealthy habits. Instead, let your detoxification program and fast be the beginning of a new, healthier lifestyle.

To make juicing a regular part of your healthy lifestyle, consume at least 8–16 ounces of juiced vegetables and fruits daily. Continue using the Green Superfood on a daily basis, too. It's about equal to getting six servings of vegetables.

In addition, keep eating lots of fruits, vegetables and whole grains as well as legumes, nuts and seeds. Eat smaller amounts of lean, free-range meats and poultry. Limit or avoid dairy. Choose skim milk products if you consume dairy. Limit or avoid processed foods. Finally, choose good fats such as extra-virgin olive oil instead of saturated and hydrogenated fats.

SHOPPING LIST

When you go to the grocery store, shop for the following organic fruits and vegetables: carrots, cabbage, apples, cucumbers, beets, celery, parsley, berries (including straw-berries, blackberries, blueberries, raspberries), lemons and limes, grapefruit, pineapple, ginger root, watermelon, garlic, greens (including spinach, collard greens, beet greens, dan-delion greens), tomatoes, sweet potatoes and dandelion root.

Add to your list any blood-type vegetables and fruit you want to try and any new, unusual fruits and vegetables with which you want to experiment.

❑ _____   ❑ _____

❑ _____   ❑ _____

❑ _____   ❑ _____

❑ _____   ❑ _____

❑ _____   ❑ _____

❑ _____   ❑ _____

❑ _____   ❑ _____

❑ _____   ❑ _____

❑ _____   ❑ _____

❑ _____   ❑ _____

❑ _____   ❑ _____

❑ _____   ❑ _____

❑ _____   ❑ _____

THE LEMONADE FAST "MASTER CLEANSE"

You may want to use a master cleanse periodically to help your body detoxify. There are several kinds available at health food stores, or you can use the following recipe to create your own: [6]

- 2 Tbsp. fresh squeezed lemon or lime juice
- 1 Tbsp. 100 percent pure maple syrup
- $\frac{1}{10}$ tsp. cayenne pepper
- 8 oz. spring water
- Liquid Stevia to taste

Mix and drink 8 to 12 glasses a day. Eat or drink nothing else except water, laxative herb tea, peppermint tea or chamomile tea.

IN CONCLUSION

Remember that your body is the temple of God. Determine to keep it strong and healthy. Continue to do periodic juice fasts every month or every two to three months, depending on your degree of toxicity or if you have a degenerative disease. You will reap a lifelong harvest of good health.

Third John 2 says, "Beloved, I wish above all things that thou mayest prosper and be in health, even as thy soul prospereth" (KJV). You will fulfill this scriptural truth in your own body and the bodies of your family members by sowing to your health and reaping the reward of divine health.

An essential part of this program is the role it plays in cleansing and restoring your body's own powerful detoxification system. I'd like to turn now and look at this amazing cleansing and purifying system God has placed in your body. By better understanding how detoxification works within you, you can be better equipped to help your body enjoy vital and life-giving toxic relief.

SEVEN

Your Champion Prize Fighter

You may be old enough to remember the garbage workers' strike in New York City. The garbage piled high along all the streets and curbs. Before long, it overflowed into the streets and littered the sidewalks. You can't imagine the smell! Before it was all over, the backlog of uncollected trash and garbage threatened to cripple the entire city and affect the health of everyone in it. What a mess!

Many of our bodies are in the same state of crisis, but we don't know it. The garbage from our diet, the garbage from our unhealthy lifestyle and the garbage from our toxic environment are crippling our entire systems to a point that degenerative disease begins.

Chemicals and toxins are everywhere. Our bodies simply cannot keep up.

Yet, even though we are bombarded by toxins without and within, our bodies are uniquely created to handle enormous amounts of toxins, poisons, germs and diseases. Your body's detoxification system is astonishingly powerful—and with the proper support and diet it is able to both detoxify and eliminate chemicals and toxins.

That's where you come in. You have it within your power to provide your incredible liver and GI tract with enough help so that they can once again function at peak efficiency. The benefits to you are unending. They include preventing and even reversing disease, having more energy, looking better, feeling better, losing weight and much more.

It's important to gain a good understanding of just what these amazing detox systems are all about. For they are your first line of defense against disease. If you don't have cancer, heart disease or another degenerative disease, these defense systems may be the reason.

The first system of toxic cleansing is your liver. It's an amazing organ that works day and night to cleanse your blood from chemicals, poisons, bacteria and any other foreign invader that comes to rob you of your good health.

To be healthy and live on this toxic planet, you must have a healthy liver. Your liver is a champion prize fighter among detox organs. You must keep it healthy and working at peak efficiency. That's why it's vital that before you begin your fast you undergo a two-week nutritional program (four weeks if you're extremely toxic) to strengthen and support your liver so it can carry out its key role in the detoxification process. (See chapter 8 for the nutritional program.)

If you were a general in the army fighting an all-out war, you wouldn't send your best, front-line troops into battle without the best weapons, uniforms and provisions. Well, because of the toxic world in which you live, your body is fighting a war every day. The good news is that it's a war that it can win. But you have an enormous part in ensuring the long-term successful outcome.

Let's look at some of the vital ways in which you can supercharge your liver's front-line defense abilities against toxins, chemicals and poisons. But first, let's get a good understanding of what this amazing front line of defense actually does for you.

YOUR BODY'S NATURAL DETOX SYSTEM

The liver weighs about five pounds and is the largest single organ and the hardest-working organ in the body. If you could look into your body right now, you would see that your liver is about the size of a football. It sits not far from your heart, which is about the size of your fist.

This amazing detox organ has many, many functions—about five hundred as a matter of fact. But it has five main functions. Let's look at them:

1 It is a major part of your body's immune defense, filtering your blood to remove toxins such as viruses, bacteria, yeast and other poisonous material.

2 It stores vitamins, minerals and carbohydrates.

3 It processes fats, proteins and carbohydrates.

4 It produces bile, a substance that breaks down fats so they can be digested.

5 It breaks down and detoxifies hormones, chemicals, toxins and metabolic waste.

HOW THIS GIANT WORKS

It's amazing how little we know about how our bodies actually work. We may understand the most complicated details about car engines and computers. Yet, few of us really comprehend the most incredible creation of all—our own human bodies. If we did, we'd be absolutely amazed.

Just how does the liver cleanse your body and keep you well? This amazing filter has three main ways to detoxify the body:

1 Filtering your blood

2 Secreting bile

3 Using a two-step enzyme process of detoxification.

Let's investigate.

YOUR GIANT FILTER

The first way is by filtering your blood. Do you have a car? The oil filter in your car filters the oil, keeping it clean so that the engine runs smoothly. But what would happen if you changed the oil without changing the oil filter? The fresh new oil would become dirty as it passed through the dirty oil filter. The liver detox program and fasting are like changing the oil filter so the liver can get caught up on its work of cleansing and detoxing the body.

Every minute, about two quarts of blood is filtered through your liver. That's an amazing amount of blood when you consider that most of our bodies have only about five quarts of blood.

If you have a swimming pool in your backyard for your kids, its filter would have to clean about half of the pool's water every minute to keep up with what your liver can do. Wow! That's how incredibly powerful this giant filter is!

When your liver is working efficiently, it is able to filter out 99 percent of the bacteria and other poisonous toxins from your blood before sending it back into circulation.

Are you the one in your family who is responsible for keeping the oil filters in your car changed? Or are you responsible to keep the air filters for your heating or air conditioning system clean? Perhaps you've been the one in charge of maintaining the filter in your backyard pool. If so, you have a pretty good idea of how much maintenance a filter requires. Any filter needs continual maintenance to keep it clean and efficient. Your liver is no different.

Think about the filthy filter that you pull out of your air conditioner, or that filthy, black oil filter you take out of your car after three thousand miles. Filters become packed with the dirt and grime they clean. And like any other filter, your liver can get overloaded with toxins.

Here are some ways that your natural filter gets overloaded with toxins:

○ From toxins in our food

○ From water with too much bacteria, chemicals, heavy metals and so forth

○ Because of digestion problems

○ From yeast and bacterial overgrowth in the small intestines

○ From food allergies

○ From parasites

○ From toxins in the air

○ From toxins in the home or workplace

○ From free radicals produced in the liver from detoxification

Like the dust and dirt that accumulate in your air filter, these toxins will eventually overwork your liver so that it may not be able to filter effectively. When this happens, your liver has to work harder and harder to keep filtering toxins. Before long it gets so overworked that it cannot function very well.

If you have ever tried to vacuum your carpet when the sweeper bag was full, then you can picture how this could happen. Now you begin to experience the symptoms of toxic overload.

WATCH FOR THE SIGNS

We doctors are always looking for signs that indicate something is going on beneath the body's surface that we can't easily see. You should learn to watch for certain signs, too. Here are some signs that will indicate to you that your body is on toxic overload: autoimmune diseases such as rheumatoid arthritis, lupus, multiple sclerosis, Crohn's disease and ulcerative colitis; osteoarthritis; chronic fatigue; chronic headaches; psoriasis; acne; food allergies; constipation; diabetes; coronary artery disease; atherosclerosis; chronic infections; recurrent infections; angina and hypertension.

If you have any of these signs of toxic overload, you will need to go on a two-week liver dietary program to build up your liver before you begin your detox fast.

WHAT ABOUT YOU?

Are you often irritable? Do you have bouts of anger and even rage? Do you have dark circles under your eyes? You may have liver toxicity. It's very common for those with a toxic liver to have bouts of anger and rage. Here are some other symptoms you should watch for:

○ Pallid skin

○ A coated tongue

○ Bad breath

○ Skin rashes

○ Poor skin tone

○ Itchy, weepy, swollen and red eyes

○ Yellow discoloration of the eyes

○ Offensive body odor

○ Itchy skin

○ Altered or bitter taste in your mouth

LIVER DETOX METHOD # 2

The filtering of blood performed by the liver is only the beginning. It is Detox Method #1. The liver also detoxifies your body by removing toxins in the "bile." This is Detox Method #2.

Every day your liver produces about a quart of bile. This substance actually helps to digest dietary fats by breaking them down so they can be used as fuel. You see, your body could never fully use the olive oil, nuts and other fatty foods you feed it without this complex method of processing it.

Not only does it break down fats, but it also breaks down fat-soluble vitamins through this same process.

A very important function of bile, however, is to eliminate poisonous toxins from your body. It becomes the vehicle for flushing them out of your body through your colon. This process starts in the liver where they pass through bile ducts, which empty into the small intestine, and are eventually eliminated through the colon. However, if you are constipated or you don't eat enough fiber or high-fiber foods, these toxins and bile may remain in the intestines too long. When this happens, the toxic poisons that should have been flushed from your body are actually reabsorbed.

In a manner of speaking, this situation is little different than when your septic system backs up, except that the toxic effect may even be worse. But the difference is that you don't notice it right away. You may not notice it for years, until disease and chronic pain begin to rob you of your freedom and vitality.

You can keep this kind of backup from taking place by making sure your diet is loaded with plenty of fiber. Such a simple solution really can spare you years of grief and pain because of degenerative illness!

If your diet lacks fiber, bile and toxins will circulate back to the liver by way of a system known as the "entero-hepatic circulation." In this system, 95 percent of bile acids and the toxins they contain are reabsorbed by a portion of the small intestines called the ileum. From here they are taken back to the liver.

The bile that is produced by the liver is actually stored in the gallbladder. The liver excretes its toxins in the bile. Bile is the fluid manufactured from three ingredients: bilirubin, lecithin and cholesterol. If these three ingredients get out of balance, such as when you have too much cholesterol, then crystals or even gallstones can form.

LIVER DETOX METHOD #3

Method number three is by far and away the most important one. This is the method of detoxing out poisons and other toxic debris. It involves a two-step process that has the same effect as changing the oil filter on your car.

This two-step process of detoxification neutralizes toxins and other chemicals and substances that need to be removed from the body. It is an absolutely phenomenal process that deep cleanses and removes most of the thousands of poisons, chemical and toxins to which we are exposed every day.

Your liver performs more than five hundred different functions, and many of them are happening at the same time. Still, this two-step filtering process is your liver's greatest and most important role. Without it, your body would suffer the same fate as your car if you never changed the oil filter. It would fill up so full of deadly poisons that you would eventually die.

Many of these chemicals are fat-soluble, which means that they can be stored in the fatty tissues of the body if the toxins are not effectively detoxified and eliminated by the liver and GI tract. These toxins can be stored for years on end and later released when you diet, exercise or perspire— but especially when you fast. Saunas and exercise that involves perspiring are also excellent ways to excrete fat-soluble toxins through the skin, which is the body's largest excretory organ.

Have you ever placed vinegar and oil in a jar and shaken them together to pour on a salad? If you let the jar sit for a few minutes, they eventually separate because oil and water don't mix.

They don't mix in your body, either. So when your body wants to remove fats or fat-soluble chemicals and toxins, it must change them into a water-soluble form to get rid of them. Your amazing liver does just that. It transforms these fat-soluble toxins and chemicals into water-soluble chemicals so they can be excreted from the body.

This two-step filtering process is simply called Phase One and Phase Two detoxification. Let's take a look at these life-saving processes.

PHASE ONE DETOXIFICATION— YOUR CHEMICAL FACTORY

Not only is your liver a giant filter, but it is also a chemical factory. Phase One detoxification involves thousands of chemical reactions. In the Phase One detoxification pathway, enzymes break down poisonous toxins. Phase One detoxification uses about fifty to a hundred different enzymes to accomplish its task.

When a toxin is processed by the Phase One detoxification system, different things can happen to it.

☼ It may become neutralized.

☼ It may be changed into a less toxic form.

☼ It may become more water soluble and then eliminated through the bile or urine.

☼ It may be transformed into an even more toxic substance that will create more free radicals.

This final result of Phase One can damage your liver. When these very toxic substances are formed, they can produce so many free radicals that they drain your liver of its antioxidants, including the vital antioxidant glutathione.

WHAT HAPPENS DURING PHASE TWO?

Phase Two detoxification kicks in when Phase One has created one of these intermediate substances. A toxic intermediate is similar to a stubborn stain that needs a second wash and rinse cycle to remove it.

These intermediate toxic compounds that have been partially detoxified by the Phase One detoxification pathways now need to be further broken down and bound to an amino acid or nutrient for Phase Two detoxification; however, the glutathione conjugation pathway is probably the most important pathway. This pathway is responsible for detoxification of approximately 60 percent of the toxins that are excreted in the bile. This pathway detoxifies toxic metals, petroleum products, many solvents, drugs such as Tylenol and penicillin, bacterial toxins and alcohol.

If too many drugs, chemicals or toxins are processed, the nutrition it takes to fuel so much detoxification gets used up. Poisonous toxins then begin to build up again. At a cellular level, it starts to look like the New York garbage strike.

EATING FOR YOUR LIVER

Since our diets often consist of processed, refined and fast foods, many Americans lack the necessary vitamins, minerals, amino acids and other nutrients the liver needs to do the job of Phase Two detoxification. When you combine poor nutrition with our overwhelming exposure to toxins, it is not difficult to see how the liver becomes overloaded and overwhelmed.

Through Phase One detoxification, your liver is able to change drugs, toxins, chemicals and hormones into intermediate compounds that are now ready to be excreted or to go through Phase Two detoxification. Phase One is similar to bagging your garbage and taking it out to the street. Phase Two is like the garbage man putting it in his garbage truck and taking it to the dump. However, for efficient Phase Two detoxification, your liver must have specific raw materials for each individual detoxification "pathway."

When large amounts of drugs, toxins or heavy metals pass through your liver, they can use up much of the store of the antioxidant glutathione. Your body has more of the powerful antioxidant glutathione than any other antioxidant—and it is probably the most important antioxidant as well. This mighty antioxidant helps the body rid itself of heavy metals such as mercury, lead and arsenic.

Too much exposure to toxic chemicals, especially heavy metals, will cause your body's glutathione levels to be depleted. A diet too low in protein, cruciferous vegetables or other sources of glutathione can also cause your body's reserves to dip too low. Here are some other factors that will drain glutathione from your body:

○ Exposure to cigarette smoke

○ Excessive exposure to pesticides

○ Excessive exposure to auto exhaust

○ Excessive exposure to paint fumes

○ Alcohol consumption

○ Excessive exercise, such as marathons

When glutathione is used up faster than it can be produced or absorbed from your diet, you become much more susceptible to cancer.

The special diet in the next chapter is designed to help you to be sure that your body has all of this powerful antioxidant it needs.

SLOWING DOWN THE PROCESS

It's essential that Phase One and Phase Two are able to move along without any hindrances. Imbalances can create problems. Taking too many medicines all at once can slow down Phase One. Toxins and even certain foods can slow down this process also. This may cause a toxic buildup or toxic overload that can damage the DNA of the liver cells.

Some medications can hinder Phase One enzymes. They include:

○ Antihistamines (Seldane and Hismanal, which have been taken off the market)

○ Ketoconazole (Nizoral, an antifungal medication)

☺ Benzodiazepenes such as Xanax, Ativan and Valium (Do not stop taking these medications, but consult your physician to see if you can be slowly weaned off them.)

So, if you have any of the symptoms of toxicity, stay away from these medications. It's important that your body's process of cleansing progress unhindered.

DETOXING TOO QUICKLY

Trouble also results when the detox process moves too quickly. When Phase One breaks down toxins so fast that Phase Two cannot process them all, those extremely poisonous intermediate toxins build up. If you remember, these intermediate toxins can be more dangerous than they were before the process began. So, you can see why it's important to keep this cleansing process moving along. Getting stalled along the way can spell disaster.

When the process gets stalled and dangerous poisons back up, enormous amounts of free radicals are released that can cause great damage, not only to the liver, but to other tissues and organs as well.

When this occurs, bile can damage the intestines and the pancreas. Free radicals can damage cells, and can even cause genetic damage, leading to cancer. Therefore, it's essential to keep these powerful detoxification phases functioning in synchrony smoothly and cleanly.

The special dietary program outlined in the following chapter will help you to do just that. This nutritional program is uniquely designed to strengthen and support your liver to prepare it for the increased role of detoxification during your fast.

IN CONCLUSION

Now you can see what a vital organ your liver is. It is the heavyweight champion of detoxification. Turn over to the next chapter to discover how you can get this fighter in shape so that it will be ready to go the distance during detox fasting.

EIGHT

A Nutritional Program for a Healthy Liver

t's impossible to get away from it. You are what you eat—especially when it comes to your physical body. And what you eat will make all the difference in maintaining your liver.

This program of cleansing and detoxification begins with a diet and regimen of supplements that you will need to take for a period of two weeks to prepare your body for a juice fast and to restore your body following the fast.

The first part of this program is dietary. The following dietary guidelines will help cleanse and support your liver before and after your detox fast. To get the optimum benefit of this plan, be careful to strictly follow these guidelines.

First, you need to change your diet and lifestyle to reduce the amount of toxins you are taking in. In addition, you will want to improve your body's ability to eliminate toxins.

ELIMINATE TOXINS

Avoid cigarette smoke, alcohol and drugs. Set a goal of decreasing your intake of all medications. If you are on prescription medicines, you must, of course, do this with your doctor's help. Except for a few medications that will be mentioned later, it is best not take any medications during your detox fast.

If you take a lot of over-the-counter medicines, consider more natural ways to treat your various medical conditions, such as using vitamins, herbs and homeopathics. In other words, if you have a neck strain from tension, consider warm baths and massages first before taking medications for neck pain. If you suffer from constipation, consider more natural ways to regulate your system, such as eating more fruit and vegetables, increasing fiber, taking magnesium, Vitamin C or other supplements before reaching for laxatives.

Just remember, be sensible. Never go off medications that you need without consulting your doctor.

Once your body is cleansed of built-up toxins, you may discover you have much less need for these medications.

MAKE LIVER-FRIENDLY DIET CHOICES

Cleaning the filter on your pool may seem more simple than maintaining your body's filter. But liver maintenance is not difficult. It can be accomplished by eating a liver-friendly diet. Therefore, make the right choices.

Here are some foods to avoid:

○ Processed foods

○ Refined foods

○ Simple sugars, including honey and maple syrup

○ Fast foods—burgers, fries, pizza, fried chicken, tacos

Decrease your consumption of the following:

○ Meat (choose extra-lean, free-range meats and poultry)

○ Decrease or avoid dairy products (choose skim milk, plain yogurt or kefir and small amounts of organic butter if you must have dairy products)

○ Saturated fats—cheese, marbled meats

Avoid these foods completely:

○ Hydrogenated and partially hydrogenated fats such as margarine

○ Deep-fried foods

○ Preserved meats

○ Fatty meats

○ Animal skins

○ Processed vegetable oils—most salad dressings (olive oil is a good choice to use)

○ Alcohol

○ Coffee

○ Colas

○ Dark teas (green tea is OK)

○ Chocolate

Choose a diet with plenty of the following:*

○ Organic fruits

○ Organic vegetables

○ Free-range meats that are organic

Eat as many raw vegetables as possible. When cooking vegetables, steam fresh vegetables instead of boiling them. Prepared fresh vegetables are always better than canned or frozen. Try preparing homemade vegetable soup, too. It's a

*For more information on this, refer to my book *Walking in Divine Health.*

delicious way to give your body a wide variety of vegetables. Just try not to overcook them, and use as many fresh, raw vegetables as possible. You may also lightly stir-fry vegetables with olive oil.

Freshly juiced vegetables and fruits are great as well. Drink a glass of freshly juiced fruits and vegetables in the morning instead of coffee.

Certain vegetables are more important than others for liver detoxification. Cruciferous vegetables are essential. Here are some that you should eat often:

- Cabbage
- Cauliflower
- Brussels sprouts
- Broccoli
- Kale
- Collard greens
- Mustard greens
- Turnips

Here's a list of other liver-friendly vegetables to eat often:

- Legumes (or all types of beans, unless you are sensitive to them)
- Beets
- Carrots
- Dandelion root
- Dandelion greens

Cruciferous vegetables contain potent phytonutrients such as indole-3-carbinol, sulforaphane and other phytonutrients, which aid the liver in detoxifying chemicals and drugs.

Broccoli sprouts usually have the highest concentration of these phytonutrients.

LIVER-FRIENDLY STARCHES

Some starches are better than others. These include:

○ Brown rice

○ Wild rice

○ Rice crackers

○ Rice pasta

○ Brown rice bread

STARCHES TO SHUN

Some starches tend to be much less liver-friendly. Starches to avoid are as follows:

○ Wheat products, including breads, bagels, crackers, pasta, chips and cereals

○ Corn products

FABULOUS LIVER-FRIENDLY FATS

Some fats are very good for your liver and for detoxification in general. Here's a list of them.

○ Extra-virgin olive oil·

○ Avocados

○ Raw, fresh nuts and seeds (avoid peanuts and cashews)

○ Flaxseed oil (but never cook with this oil)

○ Evening primrose oil

○ Black currant seed oil

○ Borage oil

○ Fish oil

BEVERAGES ARE IMPORTANT, TOO!

What you drink and how much you drink are just as important as what you eat. Here's a list of dos:

1 Drink plenty of filtered water with fresh-squeezed lemon or lime (two quarts daily).

2 Drink fresh vegetable and fruit juices.

3 Drink green tea and other herbal teas.

Drinking at least two quarts of filtered water every day will help your kidneys eliminate toxins as well.

POWERFUL DETOX PROTEINS

For protein, eating as much fatty fish in your diet as possible is best. Avoid fresh-water fish or fish from fish farms since they tend to have higher levels of PCBs, pesticides and other toxins. For more information, read *Walking in Divine Health*.

Here's a list of powerful proteins for great detoxification.

○ Salmon, 4–6 ounces

○ Mackerel, 4–6 ounces

○ Herring, 4–6 ounces

○ Halibut, 4–6 ounces

○ Free-range, extra-lean chicken, 2–4 ounces

○ Turkey, 2–4 ounces

○ Free-range, extra-lean beef, 2–4 ounces

○ One free-range egg on occasion

Having an occasional free-range egg will help supply the needed amino acids for Phase Two detoxification.

THE GOLDEN RULE OF LIVER CARE

The Golden Rule is one of the most important rules for living with others. Here's the Golden Rule of liver care: *Don't overeat.* Only eat until you are satisfied and no more. Overeating places an enormous added burden on your liver and detoxification pathways.

If you tend to be an overeater, here are some pointers that can help. Fill plates and place them on the table at dinner rather than having everyone serve himself country-style from bowls. This will help you to control portions, and it will help you to resist the temptation to eat more just because it's there in front of you. Eat slower. Chew up your food and rest between bites. Set your fork down between bites. Let your dining be an experience. Don't shovel food in nonstop like a starving man. Give your stomach a chance to find out how full it is getting before you give it more. Plan a walk right after dinner rather than sitting and visiting at the dinner table where you may be tempted to overeat. When you dine out, try not to be a charter member of the "clean plate club." Restaurant portions are too large for most people. Take half of those enormous portions home in a doggy bag for the next day, or split the meal with your spouse.

Let's turn now and look at some nutrients that are essential for your detox program.

NUTRIENTS FOR THE LIVER

These supplements should be taken to strengthen and support your liver to prepare for a detoxification fast and when coming off of a detoxification fast.

A GOOD MULTIVITAMIN/ MULTIMINERAL SUPPLEMENT

Taking a comprehensive multivitamin and mineral supplement on a daily basis is absolutely essential to promote effective liver detoxification. A good multivitamin will contain an entire array of B vitamins, which are essential for many reasons. Let's look:

○ Vitamin B_2 is used by the body in the manufacture of glutathione.

○ B_1, or thiamine, helps decrease the toxic effects of alcohol, cigarette smoking and heavy metal toxicity.

○ B_3 is used in detoxification and is required by Phase One detoxification.

○ B_5 is required for Phase One detoxification and is important for synthesizing glucuronic acid and coenzyme A, which are very important in Phase Two detoxification.

○ B_5 also helps to detoxify acetaldehyde, which is produced from alcohol and also is produced by candida overgrowth in the intestines.

○ B_6 is required for Phase One detoxification.

○ B_{12} is required for Phase One detoxification.

○ Folic acid is required for Phase One detoxification.

A good rule of thumb is that each of the above B vitamins should be present in a dose of about 50 milligrams each, except B_{12}, which should be 100 micrograms, and folic acid should be 800 micrograms.

MINERALS

A comprehensive multivitamin and mineral will contain some absolutely essential minerals for detoxing. Here are a few:

Ö Zinc

Ö Copper

Ö Manganese

You should have about 50 milligrams of zinc, 2 milligrams of copper and 2 milligrams of manganese. These three form the powerful antioxidant enzyme superoxide dismutase, which protects the liver against free radical damage.

Ö Selenium

Ö Magnesium

I recommend at least 200 micrograms of selenium and 400 miliigrams of magnesium. Selenium is part of the enzyme glutathione peroxidase, and it acts as an antioxidant. It protects cell membranes from free-radical damage. Selenium also protects the liver from the toxic effects of heavy metals such as cadmium, mercury, lead and arsenic.

Magnesium is a cofactor used in over three hundred different enzyme reactions. Magnesium also helps to manufacture DNA for protein synthesis, fatty acid synthesis and removal of toxic substances. Therefore, it is critically important for the liver to have adequate amounts of magnesium so that the liver can continue to perform its other roles of protein, carbohydrate and fat metabolism.

All of these vitamins and minerals listed above can be found in a comprehensive multivitamin such as Divine Health Whole Food Multivitamin and Mineral Supplement. (See Appendix C.)

As you can imagine by now, antioxidants are extremely important in this vital work of your liver. Making sure you have enough of them is essential. Let's look.

ANTIOXIDANTS

VITAMIN C

Vitamin C is able to raise levels of glutathione. It is also an excellent antioxidant for decreasing free radicals. In high doses, vitamin C is able to remove or chelate heavy metals such as mercury and lead.

During liver detoxification, take 1 to 2 grams of vitamin C, three times a day. However, if you begin to experience diarrhea, decrease the dose and then gradually increase it. The high dose is just for the 1–2 weeks of liver detox prior to your fast. I usually continue my patients on 1000 milligrams three times daily. I recommend Divine Health Buffered Vitamin C. (See Appendix C.)

LIPOIC ACID

Lipoic acid is a very special antioxidant that can penetrate water-soluble and fat-soluble compartments of the body and rid the body of water and fat-soluble free radicals. Lipoic acid is also able to recycle both vitamin E and vitamin C. It has been used to treat heavy metal poisoning from mercury and lead. Lipoic acid has also been used in treating liver disease.

During liver cleansing, take 100–300 milligrams of lipoic acid, two to three times a day.

VITAMIN E

Vitamin E is a fat-soluble vitamin. It actually gets incorporated into the fatty portions of cells. Here it can protect these structures from free-radical reactions, radiation, drugs and even heavy metals.

During liver detoxification, take 400 to 800 international units of vitamin E daily.

COENZYME Q_{10}

Coenzyme Q_{10}, otherwise known as CoQ_{10}, is found throughout the body. It is sometimes called "ubiquinone" since it is ubiquitous, or everywhere. It is most concentrated in the heart. This powerful antioxidant protects cell structures and other substances of the body against free-radical damage. It also protects vitamin E from oxidative damage.

Coenzyme Q_{10} is very important in energy production in the cells. It has been used to treat cardiovascular disease, including congestive heart failure, cardiomyopathy, angina and hypertension. Coenzyme Q_{10} may have a role in both cancer treatment and cancer prevention.

For detoxification, I recommend at least 100 milligrams daily with food.

Let's now look at bioflavonoids and investigate their importance to your program of detoxification.

BIOFLAVONOIDS

More than six thousand different bioflavonoids exist. These are water-soluble plant pigments that pack a powerful health punch. The most important ones for detoxification are:

○ Milk thistle (silymarin)

○ Green tea

○ Grape seed extract

○ Pine bark extract

○ Curcumin

Let's take a closer look at these.

MILK THISTLE

Milk thistle's extract, known as silymarin, is one of the most powerful protectors of the liver against free-radical damage. It also protects the liver from many different extremely toxic chemicals, including the poisonous mushroom amanita phalloides, which is actually fatal in 40 percent of the people who ingest it.

Milk thistle prevents the depletion of glutathione. Since

vast amounts of glutathione can be expended in the detoxification process, it can lead to glutathione depletion. Milk thistle will prevent this depletion during detoxification. Milk thistle can actually raise the level of glutathione in the liver up to 35 percent.

Milk thistle is the most important antioxidant to take during the detoxification fasting program.

Take 200 milligrams of milk thistle three times a day during detoxification, and drink milk thistle tea while fasting. After detoxification I recommend taking an ongoing dosage of 100 milligrams, two to three times a day, or more if desired.

GREEN TEA

As an antioxidant, green tea is two hundred times more powerful than vitamin E and five hundred times more powerful than vitamin C. Green tea is believed to block the effect of cancer-causing chemicals. It also activates detoxification enzymes in the liver, which helps defend your body against cancer.

For detoxification purposes, I recommend one cup of green tea two to three times a day. If you prefer, you may take one green tea capsule three times a day instead.

PINE BARK EXTRACT AND GRAPE SEED EXTRACT

Pine bark extract and grape seed extract are powerful bioflavonoid antioxidants. They are twenty times more powerful than vitamin C and fifty times more powerful than vitamin E as scavengers of free radicals. However, they work in water-soluble compartments of the body and move throughout the bloodstream.

These antioxidants are so powerful that they can inhibit the formation of one of the main carcinogens in tobacco smoke, which is benzopyrene.

I recommend 50–200 milligrams of grape seed extract or pine bark extract per day for detoxification purposes.

Curcumin

Curcumin is also a bioflavonoid. It is the compound that gives the common spice turmeric or Indian curry its yellow color. It has been used in China and India for thousands of years to protect the liver and to enhance bile flow. Curcumin inhibits some carcinogens from inducing cancer. Curcumin can also inhibit the cancer-causing effect of many of the cancer-inducing chemicals in cigarette smoke. Therefore, smokers or spouses of smokers who are exposed to a lot of secondhand smoke should either eat a lot of curry or should take supplements of curcumin. Turmeric or curcumin also acts as an anti-inflammatory similar to the new COX-2 inhibitors Vioxx and Celebrex.

For detoxification purposes I recommend one to two capsules of tumeric after each meal.

Amino acids are also necessary for proper detoxification. Let's look at these powerful substances.

AMINO ACIDS

The next groups of nutrients for detoxification include the amino acids.

NAC (N-ACETYL-CYSTEINE)

NAC, also known as N-acetyl-cysteine, is a stable form of the amino acid L-cysteine. NAC is easily absorbed by your body and easily converted to glutathione, so it increases the glutathione stores in your body. Approximately 60 percent of the toxins that are excreted in the bile are detoxified with the help of glutathione. That is why it is critically important to have plenty of it.

Glutathione supplements are very difficult for your body to absorb. But NAC supplements are easily absorbed and are much less expensive than glutathione. NAC is able to increase the production of glutathione.

However, too much NAC may act as a pro-oxidant and

increase free-radical activity in healthy patients. During detoxification I recommend NAC, 500 milligrams, one to two times a day.

The best way to raise glutathione levels is by taking vitamin C, milk thistle and NAC.

GLYCINE

Glycine is a non-essential amino acid, which simply means that the body produces it. It is critically important for certain Phase Two liver detox functions. In fact, it is the main amino acid used in a vital detox pathway.

People who suffer from excessive chemical exposure, hepatitis, arthritis and alcoholic hepatitis, as well as many other chronic diseases, will need supplementation with glycine.

Glycine actually performs more biochemical functions than any other amino acid. It is also required for the synthesis of bile salts. Glycine is also one of the components for the manufacturing of glutathione.

Glycine is important in detoxifying many drugs and chemicals. If the body doesn't have enough glycine, then the toxins and chemicals may not be detoxified and will probably stay in the body much longer. This can create more free radical activity and more damage.

Glycine is an inexpensive supplement that can be found in most health food stores. If you have one of the conditions listed above, take approximately 500–1000 milligrams of glycine, three times a day between meals.

GLUTAMINE

Glutamine is an amino acid that is also important in the Phase Two detoxification of the liver. It is essential for anyone who drinks excessive amounts of alcohol.

Glutamine supplementation will also help decrease intestinal permeability, a common condition in which the small intestines become inflamed by alcohol, anti-inflammatory medications, aspirin, food sensitivities, bacterial overgrowth or candidiasis. That inflammation causes the small intestine to become too permeable so that toxins and incompletely digested food particles can be absorbed from the GI tract directly into the blood and go to the liver. This puts an increased workload on the liver and further depletes it of detoxifying enzymes and antioxidants. Glutamine also helps to raise levels of glutathione in the body. Glutamine, cysteine, and glycine are converted into gluathione, which is the most important antioxidant and protector of the liver.

Take glutamine in a dose of 500–1000 milligrams three times a day, usually thirty minutes before meals during detoxification.

LIPOTROPIC SUPPLEMENTS

Lipotropic supplements are needed to promote the flow of fat and bile from the liver. Let's take a look at some of these.

LECITHIN

Lecithin is one of the best supplements to thin the bile so that toxins and chemicals can flow out of the liver more readily. Lecithin is composed of choline, inositol and linoleic acid. Choline is the main nutrient in lecithin. Choline is also found in egg yolks, soy beans, grains and nuts. By improving the flow of toxic bile from the liver during detoxification, one will be protecting the liver also.

Lecithin helps to break down fats and helps to detoxify a fatty liver.

Take at least 1000 milligrams of lecithin, three times a day during detoxification. You can take it in capsule form or granular form.

BEETS

The last lipotropic nutrient I would like to talk about is beets. Beets contain betaine, which promotes the flow of fat and bile from the liver. Betaine also protects the liver from the toxic effects of alcohol.

Betaine helps to prevent the buildup of homocysteine, which is the very toxic intermediate substance produced if you have a deficiency of the B vitamins folic acid, B_{12} and B_6.

Eat beets regularly to cleanse and support the liver, especially during detoxification, and juice beets while fasting. You may also take a beet juice extract called BetaTCP from Biotics. (See Appendix C.)

HERBS FOR DETOXING

Several herbs are very important for cleansing the liver. These include dandelion root, burdock root, red clover, ginger root and nettles. You can purchase herb teas made from these herbs to drink for liver cleansing. You can find dandelion root tea in most health food stores. Drink one of these teas one to three times a day.

CONCLUSION

Well, there you have it, a nutritional program that can get you started on the path to detoxification. As you've seen, the liver's role in detoxification is absolutely vital. However, the liver is not the only player in the game. Let's turn now and get a good understanding of how to eliminate the toxins through the GI tract.

SUMMARIZING MAIN SUPPLEMENTS

○ Comprehensive multivitamin/mineral

○ Comprehensive antioxidant formula including lipoic acid, vitamin C, vitamin E, CoQ_{10}, grape seed extract or pine bark extract and green tea (See Appendix C.)

○ Milk thistle

○ Amino acids (NAC is the most important)

○ Lipotropics–lecithin and beets

○ Detox teas, dandelion tea

NINE

"Eliminate the Negative"

Several years ago, a petite young woman named Betty*
came to my office. She had the worst case of toxicity
I've ever seen in a cancer-free person. Her skin was
ashen gray. Her long, light brown hair was thin, dull and brittle as straw. Dark black shadows encircled her sunken, lifeless
eyes. Her body looked swollen and puffy, and she complained of feeling absolutely awful and tired all the time.
Although only twenty-eight years of age, she was in quite a
lot of pain from rheumatoid arthritis and looked much older
than her age.

I realized in just a few minutes of examining her that if she
didn't begin to detoxify, she'd probably be back to see me
with possibly another autoimmune disease, cancer or some
other degenerative disease.

As I questioned her about her lifestyle, Betty painted a picture of a fairly ordinary American diet. It was unhealthy, centered around pizza, Big Macs, sodas and fries with very little
fruit and vegetables. She drank little water, and instead polished off an entire pot of coffee every day, which she prepared

---

*Fictitious character

with lots of sugar and heavy cream. She was, no doubt, somewhat dehydrated. But even this awful diet couldn't totally explain her toxic state.

I probed further, asking about the functioning of her GI tract and colon. As she shared her story, I began to understand why she was so ill.

She traveled often, and each time she left town she'd become a bundle of nerves. As a result, her colon would seemingly just stop. She would go for days on end without a bowel movement—sometimes for an entire week.

Because of her diet of fats and refined sugar and her lack of adequate water and fiber, her food would sit in her colon while many of the dangerous toxins in the stool were reabsorbed back into her body. She was in trouble from toxicity, and if she didn't begin to have daily bowel movements, she would eventually be even sicker. This young woman desperately needed toxic relief.

This woman's toxicity wasn't due to her liver. As a matter of fact, her liver seemed surprisingly strong considering the state of her health. No, her toxicity was mainly a result of an unusually slow and poorly cared for intestinal tract.

This young woman's condition is not at all uncommon, which is why we must carefully examine the main avenue for elimination, which is the intestinal tract or small intestines and colon.

Finding toxic relief is a little like the old song that tells us we have to "eliminate the negative." In order for your body to efficiently eliminate its toxic buildup of chemicals, toxic fat and other poisons, you must first get your intestinal tract in top condition. Without both a healthy, well-functioning liver and a healthy intestinal tract, your body will continue to labor under a dangerous burden of toxins.

The liver processes and detoxifies the toxins. However the intestinal tract is responsible for removing the majority of the toxins. The liver excretes the toxins through the bile. If the bowel function is sluggish or if there is insufficient fiber in your diet, the toxins will usually be reabsorbed by the intestines and further burden the liver and entire body with excessive toxins.

Before you start this program of detoxification, you will need to get your colon in shape. So, let's get started.

YOUR FIRST LINE OF DEFENSE

Every team has its first team player who seems to dominate the game while others sit on the bench waiting for their special skills to be called upon. Your intestinal tract never sits out the game. It is definitely a powerful player in your defense against toxicity.

It's important to have a good understanding of how this amazing system works. Let's look.

A LOOK INSIDE

Imagine that your skin suddenly turned to glass so that you could see everything going on inside of you. You would quickly see that your intestinal tract is, stated simply, a long tube. As a matter of fact, it is a continuous tube that's more than twenty feet long. It connects your entire digestive system together. Your food enters the tube on one end and exits on the other.

In between, your food undergoes a miracle of processing. The mouth starts the process and connects with the esophagus. The esophagus connects with the stomach. The stomach connects with the small intestines. The small intestines connect with the large intestines, and the large intestines connect to the rectum and finally end at the anus. If digestion and elimination proceed smoothly and unhindered, then toxins are eliminated daily, and good health is achieved.

DIGESTION AND TOXICITY

Poor digestion and elimination, as in Betty's case, is one of the main causes of toxicity in your body. Digestion actually begins when your brain signals that your body needs food. For instance, it's nearing lunch time, and you start thinking about the wonderful colorful salad and whole-grain sandwich that you packed yourself for lunch. Your brain signals your digestive tract to begin producing the necessary enzymes and components for digestion.

The next step occurs when you smell and see food. You open your lunch box and smell the delicious salad and sandwich, the fresh garlic and parsley. Your mouth begins to water. Sight and smell stimulate your salivary glands to produce saliva. Saliva contains the enzyme amylase, which breaks down starches.[1] Saliva contains epidermal growth factor, which is produced in the salivary glands. It helps to stimulate the growth of cells in the liver.

The sight, smell and taste of the food trigger the process of digestion so that the stomach is prepared when the food arrives. The digestion of food in the stomach usually takes between one and four hours. A healthy stomach has a pH between 1.5 and 3.0 due to hydrochloric acid, which is secreted by the stomach. Hydrochloric acid is strong enough to burn a hole through the carpet or to melt the iron in a nail. You can see how this powerful acid forms the first line of defense against bacteria, parasites and germs. Its acidic pH makes it a strong sterilization system against such invaders from our food.

You've enjoyed chewing and swallowing your satisfying salad and sandwich. It has traveled to your stomach where this powerful acid breaks it down.

DILUTING YOUR STOMACH ACID

It's important that stomach acid retain its full strength. However, many people dilute this acid by chewing their food only a couple of times and washing it down with a giant gulp of ice-cold soda or iced tea.

Cold foods and cold beverages decrease circulation in the stomach and intestines and slow down the digestive process. Cold drinks also wash out digestive enzymes. Ideally, it's best to drink your beverages about thirty minutes before eating a meal. The best beverage to consume is filtered water at room temperature. You may drink 4 ounces of water with a meal.

Poor posture also affects digestion. While eating, try to sit up straight to take the weight and the burden off the digestive tract.

THE PATH YOUR FOOD TRAVELS

Now, your digested salad and sandwich leaves your stomach. It exits in a semi-liquid food form called *chyme.* Then it moves into the small intestine, which measures about eighteen to twenty-three feet in the average adult. That is about four times longer than you are tall.

The small intestine is divided into three sections. The *duodenum* is the first area of the small intestine that receives the partially digested salad and sandwich from the stomach. Then your lunch travels to the *jejunum* where most of the nutrients are absorbed into the blood. Your delicious and nourishing sandwich completes its visit in the small intestines in the *ileum,* the third and final portion of the small intestines. Here the remaining nutrients from your lunch are absorbed before it moves into the large intestines.

For the nutrients from your lunch to be absorbed into your body, they must first come in contact with a sea of special cells in your intestines. These cells contain thousands of tiny fingerlike projections called *villi.* About twenty thousand villi are found on every square inch of your small intestines. These little fingers sway back and forth constantly, stirring up your now liquefied lunch to remove its nutrients.

Your sandwich has now been broken down into such small particles that they can pass into the villi where they can be taken up and absorbed by very small blood vessels called capillaries. These capillaries transport your lunch to your liver. All the nutrients from your sandwich are absorbed through the intestinal walls. Minerals are absorbed mainly in the duodenum. Carbohydrates, proteins and water-soluble vitamins are absorbed mainly in the jejunum, and fat and fat-soluble vitamins are absorbed mainly in the ileum.

GETTING RID OF THE WASTE

Now your sandwich can be used to fuel your body in the many thousands of wonderful ways in which the vitamins, minerals and other nutrients it contains can do. But if you've ever built a fire in your fireplace or driven behind a bus, you know that fuel cannot be burned without also creating smoke, or waste products. Your body's elimination is similar in that the intestine absorbs nutrients and excretes the waste.

The waste products of this process are then propelled mainly into the colon. There they usually remain for one to two days, and in some patients seven days or longer. They are then expelled by a bowel movement. The last few inches of the colon make up the rectum, which is a storage site for solid waste. The waste is then expelled through the anal opening.

The first half of the colon absorbs the fluids from this waste and recycles them into your bloodstream. The second half of your colon condenses the waste into feces. It also secretes mucus, which binds the substances together and lubricates them to protect the colon and ease its passage.

There you have it! The entire GI system of taking in the nutrients your body needs and excreting the waste.

Of the two to two and a half gallons of food and liquids taken in by the average adult each day, only about twelve ounces of waste enters into the large intestine. Feces is made up of about three-quarters water. The remainder is protein, fat, undigested food, roughage, dried digestive juices and cells shed by the intestines along with dead bacteria.

When this system of expulsion works quickly and efficiently, toxins are expelled without the opportunity for your body to reabsorb them. But when your diet is made up of too many refined sugars and processed foods, you can throw this amazingly efficient process into a tailspin. Toxins can actually sit in your colon for days on end where they are constantly being reabsorbed by your body. When this situation occurs over a long period of time, your body, and especially your fatty tissues, can become full of toxins.

NATURAL DIET VS. AMERICAN DIET

Years ago, Dr. Dennis Burkett, a famous English physician, examined the digestive differences of rural Africans who ate a natural, fiber-rich diet that was packed with fresh fruits and vegetables, complex carbohydrates and little meat. He compared the diet of the naval officers whose diet was basically meat, white flour and sugar, similar to the basic American diet.[2]

The Africans had large, effortless stools approximately eighteen to thirty-six hours after they ate. In comparison, the English naval officers experienced small, difficult, compact, hard stools seventy-two to one hundred hours after eating.[3]

The naval officers also developed hemorrhoids, anal fissures, varicose veins, diverticulitis, diverticulosis, thrombophlebitis, gallbladder disease, appendicitis, hiatal hernia, irritable bowel syndrome, obesity, high cholesterol, coronary artery disease, high blood pressure, diabetes, hypoglycemia, colon polyps and colon and rectal cancers.

The Africans only experienced these things after they converted to a British diet consisting mainly of meat, white flour and sugar.

As you can see, what you eat makes all the difference in the world when it comes to healthy and efficient GI elimination.

Not only does diet play an enormous role, your GI tract must face challenges from many other factors that can significantly influence how well it digests and detoxifies your food. Let's take a look at a few of them.

WHAT'S AFFECTING YOU?

The efficiency of your GI tract is being challenged every day. One of those challenges comes from a deficiency of those incredibly powerful digestive juices.

If you're over fifty years old, you may be among the many middle-aged individuals who begin to experience a reduction in the hydrochloric acid that is so essential to digestion. When the levels of this acid become depleted, digestive problems follow.

If stress plays a major role in your life, you probably don't need me to tell you that it affects digestion. It's not unusual for stressed-out individuals to have stomach medications strewed all around their workplace and car.

If you are stressed, you are probably not only deficient in hydrochloric acid, but you may be deficient in pancreatic enzymes as well. The lack of these vital pancreatic enzymes causes poor digestion of proteins, fats and carbohydrates. When this happens, bits of partially digested food can putrefy and travel through your GI tract, leading to bacterial overgrowth in the small intestines, food allergies and so forth.

As you can imagine, food that is not completely digested creates an onslaught of problems for your body. An enormous stream of dangerous toxins is created that can overload and overwhelm your liver. Partially digested proteins can be absorbed directly into your bloodstream, causing painful food allergies. Partially digested food particles also may lead to the overgrowth of unfriendly bacteria, which may produce endotoxins and other dangerous toxins in the GI tract.

RELAX . . . BREATHE . . . TAKE A MINUTE

Don't eat when you're stressed. Before you pick up your fork, take a brief moment to relax a bit. It's extremely important. If you tend to eat on the run or when you're upset, angry or fearful, such negative emotions will have an effect. They will stimulate the sympathetic nervous system, which will result in a decreased secretion of hydrochloric acid. This, in turn, reduces your secretions of pancreatic enzymes, making it very difficult to digest food.

Therefore, when you sit down to eat, take time to thank God and to meditate on all His goodness and provision. Release any negative emotions, bless the food and then begin to eat.[4] Chew your food thoroughly. This is important. Each bite should be chewed twenty to thirty times to mix enough saliva thoroughly with your food.

OVERLOADING

When your computer gets overloaded with files, programs and unnecessary junk, what happens? It goes slower and slower until it finally stops working altogether. Your GI tract may do the very same thing.

When people overeat and stuff themselves until they are full, they put an enormous strain on the digestive tract. And it's even worse if you overeat late at night before bedtime when the digestive system needs to rest.

INTESTINAL PERMEABILITY

The small intestine functions as an organ of digestion and absorption. It also functions as a barrier to keep your body from absorbing toxic materials and large molecules of undigested food.

A healthy small intestine allows absorption of some

substances—such as triglycerides from the digestion of fats, sugars from the digestion of carbohydrates, amino acids and di- and tri-peptides from the digestion of proteins. But it seals out compounds that would likely cause harm, such as partially digested bits of food, toxins and heavy metals.

Nevertheless, if you consume too much alcohol or if you take anti-inflammatory medicines or aspirin, they can irritate and inflame the lining of your intestines. This can lead to microscopic openings and holes in the small intestine. These holes will allow partially digested foods to pass directly through the intestinal wall into the blood stream. This is called increased intestinal permeability.

It can also cause food allergies or food sensitivities, inflammatory bowel disease such as ulcerative colitis, Crohn's disease, celiac disease, rheumatoid arthritis, psoriasis, schizophrenia and chronic skin problems.

Increased intestinal permeability allows undigested or partially digested food molecules, bacteria and bacterial toxins, yeast, yeast toxins, heavy metals and food antigens as well as other toxic substances to leak into the bloodstream. These toxins are then free to go directly into the liver. There, they wreak havoc, undermining detoxification and triggering the release of free radicals, which damage the liver as well as other organs and tissues throughout the body.

THE EFFECTS OF FOOD ALLERGIES

A main cause of increased intestinal permeability is food allergies and sensitivities. Common food allergies include allergies to egg, dairy products, wheat and other grains such as rye, barley and oats. The main protein that people are sensitive to in these grains is gluten, which is found in breads, crackers, pasta, all kinds of flour such as rye, barley, wheat and oat flour, gravies and many soups, bread crumbs, pies and cakes.

WATCH FOR THESE SYMPTOMS

Increased intestinal permeability is usually present in the following diseases: chronic fatigue, fibromyalgia, migraine headaches, eczema, hives, psoriasis, Crohn's disease, ulcerative colitis, celiac disease, rheumatoid arthritis, lupus, schizophrenia, autism and attention-deficit hyperactivity disorder.

If you suspect this might be an issue for you, try going on a vegetarian diet in addition to the detoxification fasting program in this book. If you are sensitive to gluten, select another form of grain for your daily diet, such as brown rice bread, millet bread, quinoa, kamut or amaranth. Buckwheat is also gluten-free, so you can still have buckwheat pancakes.

REPAIRING YOUR INTESTINES

To repair your small intestines, you must improve your digestion. You should also reinoculate the bowel with friendly bacteria (we will discuss this later.) Bowel transit time must be improved. Decrease stress, especially when eating, by eating in a relaxed, peaceful atmosphere.

Do this on a regular basis daily. Vegetarians usually have a healthy GI tract, but the majority of Americans do not and are in a desperate need for repair of the GI tract.

Supplements to help repair the GI tract

○ L-glutamine is an amino acid used to feed the cells of the small intestines. I recommend taking 500–1000 milligrams of L-glutamine thirty minutes before eating your meals for at least three months if you have increased intestinal permeability. If you have Crohn's disease, colitis, celiac disease and so forth, you may need to take this for a year or longer. To find out if you have increased intestinal permeability, see a nutritional doctor or have your doctor order Intestinal Permeability Testing. (See Appendix C.)

Ö Another nutrient that is extremely effective to the GI tract is gamma-oryzanol. This is found in brown rice. Eat plenty of brown rice, brown rice bread, rice bran or rice bran oil. Or you may take gamma-oryzanol in pill form, 100 milligrams three times a day. Again I recommend the tablet thirty minutes before meals for three months, or just eat plenty of brown rice.

Ö DGL is another supplement that can help. It is actually a kind of licorice that helps to heal the GI tract. It is best to take a chewable form (approximately 380 milligrams) three times a day, thirty minutes before meals.

Ö Finally, aloe vera juice soothes the lining of the stomach and intestines. It can be taken several times during the day.

For the majority of patients, L-glutamine, 500 milligrams, or one to two tablets thirty minutes before meals for three months is adequate to repair the GI tract. The other supplements should be added if you are not improving.

In addition, stop drinking alcohol, avoid aspirin and avoid anti-inflammatory medicines such as Advil. Identify all your food allergies and avoid those food or follow a rotation diet.

The intestinal lining is one of the fastest healing tissues in your body. As a matter of fact, it can be replaced approximately every six to ten days. For more information on this topic I recommend my booklet *The Bible Cure for Allergies*.

GOOD BACTERIA, BAD BACTERIA AND YEAST

About a hundred trillion bacteria reside in the large bowel, weighing in at about three pounds. More than four hundred different species of bacteria live there. Fortunately, most of these bacteria are extremely beneficial; you wouldn't want to try to live without them. They are responsible for many different functions, such as synthesizing vitamins and breaking down toxins. They also digest fiber by changing it into short chain fatty acids that provide the main nourishment for your colon's cells.

BACTERIA AND YOUR IMMUNE SYSTEM

Believe it or not, most of your entire immune system—about 60 percent—is located in the lining of the small intestines. Good bacteria improve your immune response. Bad bacteria, of course, do not. So, there's a very delicate, extremely important balance of power that must be maintained at all times.

It's really not much different from the balance of power that exists between the branches of our government.

The United States Supreme Court, the president and the Congress all share the power in our country. The system is set up so that no one branch is more powerful than the others. This careful and delicate balance has made it possible for us to enjoy the most powerful and influential government system in the entire world. But what would happen if an evil president got into office who decided to take over the military and overthrow the other two branches? We'd have anarchy, and our form of government would be destroyed.

Well, when the balance of government in your GI tract is overrun by bad bacteria and yeast, anarchy and chaos reign in your body, too.

This kind of chaos can happen with repeated or prolonged use of antibiotics. Overuse of antibiotics kills the harmful bacteria, but it kills the good bacteria, too. Under normal conditions, good bacterial colonies, bad bacterial colonies and yeast colonies exist together in a balance of power. Both the yeast and bad bacteria are held in check by the good bacteria.

But when overuse of antibiotics kills both the good and bad bacteria, the yeast can start to grow so rapidly in the small and large intestines that the yeast grows out of control. Yeast overgrowth may be associated with many different diseases and symptoms such as psoriasis, eczema, hives, diarrhea, bloating, gas and other symptoms.

If you use antibiotics too often or for too long, eventually the bad bacteria in your intestines may actually become resistant to them. When this occurs, bad, or pathogenic, bacteria may also grow out of control.

When these bacteria run rampant in your body, they can create poisons called endotoxins that can damage and destroy the protective coverings (membranes) of cells. This leads to even more leakage of food across your intestinal lining, resulting in more food allergies, liver toxicity and eventually systemic disease.

COUNTERFEIT PROTEINS RUNNING AMUCK

This overgrowth of dangerous pathogenic bacteria in your intestines can also fool your system and wreak untold damage. It does this through "antigenic mimicry," which is simply when proteins from intestinal bacteria are absorbed right into the bloodstream by increased intestinal permeability. The intestinal bacteria have proteins that appear to the immune system as being very similar to human protein. That's why it's call mimicry. These bacterial proteins actually mimic or counterfeit true proteins.

That may not seem so dangerous to you, but these proteins were never meant to enter directly into your blood. Because these proteins are very similar to human protein, they may actually confuse the immune system into attacking itself. The immune system will finally recognize the proteins as counterfeit and form antibodies against them to destroy them, but because the proteins mimic human proteins, the antibodies also lead to inflammation of human tissue such as joint tissue.

PARTIALLY DIGESTED FOOD

Not only can the bacteria mimic true proteins, they can also cause fermentation in your small intestines—just the way that apple cider ferments. Have you ever bought a gallon of apple cider in the fall, only to have it ferment in your fridge? What happened to it when it did? It turned into an alcoholic beverage and released lots of gasses and other toxins in the process.

Think about two to three pounds or even more of bacteria overgrowth in your small intestines fermenting and causing the partially digested food to ferment and putrefy. This putrefaction creates substances called indoles, skatols and amines, substances that can be measured in a urine indican test.

Bad bacteria also can produce enzymes that can break down your bile into toxins that can promote the development of cancer. Bacterial enzymes can also inactivate your own digestive enzymes, causing impaired digestion, malabsorption, diarrhea, bloating and gas.

FINDING FRIENDLY BACTERIA

Good bacteria, or friendly bacteria, are the lactobacilli and bifido bacteria. These GI-friendly organisms preserve the balance of power and form the defense against the rampant overgrowth of bad bacteria and yeast. Therefore, they keep poisonous toxins at bay. Beneficial bacteria also help prevent damage to the lining of the GI tract, thus maintaining normal intestinal permeability. They also prevent the growth of bacteria that produce the dangerous enzymes that promote cancer. In addition, these friendly bacteria secrete chemicals that kill the bad, or pathogenic, bacteria.

Good bacteria, called lactobacillus acidophilus, are normally found in the small intestines. Bifido bacteria are normally found in the large intestines.

Food for good bacteria, called fructo-oligosaccharides (FOS), are complex sugars that are found in high amounts in Jerusalem artichokes. FOS encourages the growth of the good bacteria and discourages the growth of the harmful bacteria. I recommend good bacteria daily, either in capsule or powder form if one desires to keep a healthy GI tract.

ACIDOPHILUS AND BIFIDO BACTERIA

If you are taking antibiotics, or if you have any of the symptoms of increased intestinal permeability, take at least three billion colony-forming units of both acidophilus and bifido bacteria every day. Keep these products in your refrigerator. (See Appendix C.)

If you have diseases associated with increased intestinal permeability, you should be on these supplements a minimum of three months and preferably indefinitely. Anyone who wants to maintain a healthy GI tract should take them regularly.

FOS

In addition, take at least 1000–3000 milligrams a day of FOS to feed the friendly bacteria. Take these at the same time that you take the acidophilus and bifidus. It is best to take all of these between meals. (See Appendix C.)

YOGURT

Many people believe that they can get enough beneficial bacteria from eating yogurt. However, many yogurts that claim they have live bacteria really do not. In addition, many yogurts contain lactobacillus bulgaricus, which only lives in the intestines for about two weeks. Therefore, I strongly suggest that you not try to rely on this method alone in supplying your intestines with friendly bacteria.

LACTOBACILLUS PLANTARUM

When you take antibiotics, you should also continue using supplements of lactobacillus acidophilus and bifidus with FOS for about a month after stopping the antibiotics. If you must take antibiotics over an extended period of time, take lactobacillus plantarum for a month also. This is the only lactobacillus that is not killed by antibiotics. Take one to two capsules a day. You will find this at a health food store.

PARASITES THAT PLUNDER

Imagine having a large tick attached to your arm that continually sucks the blood out of your body. It lives there constantly, sapping your strength and injecting poisons into your skin that make you ill. On a molecular level, that's what microscopic parasites do.

If you think that the only people who get parasites are those who travel and live in exotic, Third World countries, you're wrong. Fact is, you may have parasites living inside your body right now!

There are three classes of parasites. Parasites are simply microorganisms that live off their host (you) and eventually cause damage to the host. Parasitic infections are fairly common here in the United States. In fact, the majority of the population of the world is colonized with parasites. That means you probably have had them at some time in your life and may have them right now!

Let's take a look at these unwelcome visitors.

THE PROTOZOA

Three main groups of parasites exist. The first are one-celled organisms called protozoa. They include amoebas, giardia, cryptosporidium and blastocystis.

Giardia thrives in many of the lakes and streams throughout the United States, and it is often blamed for small outbreaks of diarrhea. When ingested, this parasite takes up residence in the

148

small intestine, creating damage that leads to increased intestinal permeability. In fact, giardia can so damage the small intestine that, even after it has been eradicated, it can take months to heal. I had a giardia infection after skiing on a lake. Not long ago, I went waterskiing with my son, Kyle, who is an excellent "wake boarder." I decided to give it a try.

I got out there on this little wake board and tried to get up, but it didn't work. My wife was driving the boat, and it seemed as if I were drinking half the water in the lake. It was embarrassing. I tried again and again until I had blisters on my hands, and finally said, "Give me the skis!" My son still laughs about it.

About four days later I felt this little gurgle in my stomach. It became worse and turned into diarrhea. It would occur one day, be gone the next, and then it would return. Finally, I checked myself and found I had giardia, a microscopic parasite that lives in the small intestines. It is common in the lakes of Central Florida.

I treated myself with herbs, and the condition cleared within two weeks.

In the 1990s the parasite *cryptosporidium* contaminated the water supply of Milwaukee, causing the largest epidemic of diarrhea in United States history. Over a hundred deaths occurred, and over four thousand people developed diarrhea.

Blastocystis is another protozoa that commonly causes diarrhea. Other symptoms that one has when infested with this parasite include bloating, flatulence and explosive, foul-smelling diarrhea.

Amoebas also cause diarrhea. They can so damage the lining of your intestines that they create leaky gut, burdening your liver.

THE WORMS (HELMINTHS)

The second group of parasites is classified as the helminths, which are worms. These include roundworms, hook worms, thread worms, tape worms, whip worms and pin worms.

THE ARTHROPODS

The third group is the arthropods, which include ticks, mites, lice and so on.

THE GIFT OF GARLIC

If you suspect that you may be infested with parasites from your drinking water or other means, supplementing with garlic can help.

Garlic is a member of the allium family, which also includes onions, scallions and leeks. Among these four, garlic contains the highest concentration of this powerful substance. Garlic has enormous powers to fight parasite infestations in your GI tract. It also kills bacteria, yeast and viruses.

I recommend approximately 500 milligrams of garlic, two tablets, three times a day. You may take this is you have diarrhea that has persisted longer than a few days. If diarrhea persists, see your physician and have a stool specimen from three different stools examined for ova and parasites. Also have a giardia antigen test and a stool culture.

Other herbs, including oil of oregano, black walnut, artemesia, pumpkin seed, cloves and grapefruit seed, are beneficial for parasitic infections. Many products have a mixture of the herbs listed above.

THE CURSE
OF CONSTIPATION

As we saw earlier in this chapter, constipation is part of the price we pay in this society for our unhealthy diet. The pharmaceutical industry is making a fortune on our addiction to sugar and refined and processed foods and on our need for laxatives, antacids and medications for bloating and gas.

Normal bowel transit time is approximately twenty to thirty hours. If your diet has plenty of fiber, your stools will be soft but formed. You will also have regular bowel movements—

about one, two or even three times a day.

A loose stool indicates intestinal irritation. It could be caused by a bacterial or viral infection, increased intestinal permeability, allergies, parasitic infections, yeast overgrowth, malabsorption or poor digestion.

Normally, movements should occur about twenty to thirty minutes after eating. Under ideal circumstances, you should have one after every meal.

LAXATIVES

Avoid using over-the-counter chemical and herbal laxatives, for these may lead to a dependency on the laxative. Osmotic laxatives such as magnesium sulfate, magnesium citrate, magnesium glycinate and magnesium aspartate are much safer alternatives. Many people are actually deficient in magnesium. Osmotic laxatives simply draw water into the colon and make the stool soft. They usually do not irritate the bowels.

VITAMIN C

Taking higher doses of buffered vitamin C can also prevent constipation as well as provide antioxidant protection. I recommend 1000–2000 milligrams of buffered vitamin C, two to three times daily, even when off the detoxification program. Everyone should take vitamin C, but those constipated usually need more. (See Appendix C.)

CHLOROPHYLL DRINKS

A chlorophyll drink such as Divine Health Green Superfood contains wheat grass, barley grass, alfalfa, spirulina, chlorella and blue-green algae. These powerful foods are full of phytonutrients and magnesium, which help to cleanse the bowels and prevent constipation.

Take one scoop each morning. Mix it with pink grapefruit juice for a delicious energy drink. If you are constipated, you may drink it two times daily. However, don't drink it in the evening or too late in the afternoon or it may give you too much energy and keep you awake. If you are still constipated, take all three supplements (magnesium, vitamin C and Green Superfood) until the bowels are regulated.

THREE MAIN FACTORS

All of these supplements are very helpful for constipation, but equally important factors for regularity include the following:

1 Drinking enough water—at least two quarts of filtered water a day

2 Regular exercise

3 A high-fiber diet with at least 30 to 35 grams of fiber per day

FANTASTIC FIBER

Fiber is fantastic for your healthy GI tract. It acts like a broom, sweeping the colon lining, eliminating the toxins and binding the toxins in the bile so that they cannot be reabsorbed back into your body. All of this activity is critically important in preventing disease. High-fiber diets also reduce the level of circulating estrogens by binding them and preventing them from being reabsorbed and recirculated through the liver.

Most of the chemicals that have been detoxified by the liver are contained in the bile, which is then dumped into the intestinal tract. This, as you know, is a major part of your body's detoxification process. But if your GI tract doesn't have enough fiber or is constipated, then much of that toxic bile will be reabsorbed back into your body. That's why it's so important to get plenty of fiber every day through your diet and to supplement with fiber regularly as well so that the toxins in your body will be bound and excreted. This will dramatically reduce your body's toxic burden. Let's take a look at this wonderful natural detoxifier.

NATURE'S DETOXIFIER

Most of your fiber should come from your diet. Eat plenty of raw fruits, raw vegetables, whole grains, beans, legumes and seeds.

Fiber comes in two varieties: water-soluble, which means they can dissolve in water, and that which is insoluble in water. Foods high in soluble fiber include oats, oat bran, guar gum, carrots, beans, apples, ground flaxseeds, psyllium and citrus pectin. Foods high in insoluble fiber include wheat bran, most root vegetables, celery and the skins of fruits. Soluble fiber feeds the intestinal bacteria—especially the good bacteria. It also provides nourishment to the cells of the colon.

Intestinal bacteria causes soluble fiber to ferment and form short-chain fatty acids. This, in turn, nourishes the cells of the large intestine. These short-chain fatty acids help to prevent the growth of yeast and harmful bacteria. However, if you eat too much soluble fiber, such as too many beans or too much guar gum, you can develop an overgrowth of intestinal bacteria along with excessive bloating, gas and abdominal discomfort.

Soluble fiber helps to lower cholesterol, control blood sugar and create a sensation of fullness so that you will be less likely to overeat.

Insoluble fiber, on the other hand, inactivates many intestinal toxins. It also helps to prevent harmful bacteria and parasites from attaching themselves to the wall of your intestines by acting like a sweeping broom.

FIBER FOODS

Since both forms of fiber are very beneficial, I strongly recommend that you eat food that contains a mixture of soluble and insoluble fibers. Rice bran, oat bran, legumes such as beans and peas, apples, pears and berries contain both sources of fiber.

I do not recommend wheat bran since so many people are sensitive to the protein in wheat (gluten). Gluten-sensitive individuals may also need to avoid oat bran since oats also contain gluten but not as much as wheat products. If you suffer with increased intestinal permeability and food allergies, eat plenty of rice bran and brown rice.

MICROCRYSTALLINE CELLULOSE

Another excellent form of insoluble fiber includes microcrystalline cellulose. You can get this from a health food store or a nutritional doctor. Since many soluble fibers can produce bloating and bacterial overgrowth, I routinely use microcrystalline cellulose. Since it is an insoluble fiber and does not contain any wheat products, it tends to be tolerated even by those with sensitive GI tracts.

FLAXSEED

Flaxseed, freshly ground in a coffee grinder, is one of the best ways to get your daily fiber. Simply put one tablespoon in a coffee grinder, and then pour the ground seeds into a smoothie or sprinkle it on your oatmeal, salad or on any other food. It is good to take this two to three times throughout the day.

Flaxseeds contain lignans, which not only help to relieve hot flashes in menopausal women, but also have antifungal, antibacterial and antiviral activity. Lignan also blocks the activity of the enzyme that converts other hormones into estrogen.

CITRUS PECTIN

Another very important fiber is citrus pectin. It is a water-soluble fiber that comes from the cell walls of citrus fruits. Animal studies have shown that modified citrus pectin inhibited the metastatic spread of cancer. In one study, the metastatic spread of cancer was reduced more than 80 percent![5]

Be cautious with guar gum. It is a soluble fiber that may cause an overgrowth of intestinal bacteria.

Take fiber each morning when you get up and again before you go to bed at night. Freshly ground flaxseed mixed with Green Superfood is one of my favorite ways to start a day.

IN CONCLUSION

Your amazing body is not only designed to detoxify itself, but to heal itself as well. And just as you can play a significant role in helping and supporting your body's own abilty to detoxify itself, you can also do the same with healing.

Let's turn and take a look at how detox fasting can play an exciting and powerful role in your body's process of healing.

SUMMARIZING MAIN SUPPLEMENTS

- L-glutamine, 500–1000 milligrams thirty minutes before meals
- Lactobacillus acidophilus and bifidus with FOS, 1 teaspoon two times a day (See Appendix C.)
- Fiber such as ground flaxseeds, 1 tablespoon two times a day
- Green Superfood, 1 scoop upon awakening

TEN

Finding Healing Through Fasting

At the age of forty-two, Rev. George Malkmus learned that he had developed colon cancer. Having watched his mother suffer and die from cancer, he determined he would not go the same route. Dr. Malkmus, a Baptist pastor, turned to his friend, evangelist Lester Roloff. Evangelist Roloff advised him not to go the medical route of chemotherapy, radiation and surgery for his cancer, but to change his diet to raw fruits and vegetables and drink a lot of freshly juiced carrot juice. Malkmus took his advice and changed his diet from a diet full of meat and cooked, processed food with an abundance of desserts to a diet of raw fruits and vegetables with one to two quarts of freshly juiced carrot juice a day. In less than a year his tumor had disappeared.

Fortunately, George Malkmus discovered his cancer at a point where he was able to reverse it with nutrition and detoxification. Through diet and detoxification his blood pressure went down, his allergies vanished and a host of other chronic complaints simply went away. That was more than twenty years ago. Today he remains as strong and healthy as ever and completely convinced that there is toxic relief.[1]

Unfortunately, not all cancers respond as his did. Therefore I recommend that patients use a comprehensive approach and seek medical opinions from both conventional medicine and nutritional doctors.

The story of George Malkmus is not uncommon. I believe that many diseases are the direct result of an excessive buildup of these toxins. I have seen this in patients with psoriasis, lupus and rheumatoid arthritis.

Here are some other diseases that are often directly linked to a buildup of toxins:

○ Food and environmental allergies

○ Asthma

○ Headaches

○ Fatigue

○ Fibromyalgia

○ Chronic back pain

○ Eczema, chronic acne and other skin conditions

○ Insomnia

○ Depression

○ Irritable bowel syndrome

○ Decreased sex drive

○ Menstrual problems

○ Abdominal bloating

○ Belching

○ Gas

○ Memory loss

○ Chronic diarrhea

○ Crohn's disease

○ Ulcerative colitis

○ Atherosclerosis

○ Hypertension

○ Obesity

○ Constipation

○ Angina

○ Multiple sclerosis

○ Coronary artery disease

○ Cancer

○ Mental illness

○ Diabetes

Now remember, whenever you are sick or diseased, your body is signaling you that it is time to rest from work. With many diseases, it's also trying to tell you to rest from foods that are difficult to digest. So instead of drinking coffee and eating foods high in sugar and caffeine, which may help you to keep on working, take a lesson from the animals.

When animals are sick, they go to a secluded place near a source of water. There, they rest, drink water and fast. Likewise, when we are sick with a temporary or chronic illness, we should also rest and fast with juices to nourish our bodies and support the liver as it works hard to detoxify from our illness.

Fasting does not only prevent sickness. If done correctly, fasting holds amazing healing benefits to those of us who suffer illness and disease. From colds and flu to heart disease, fasting is a mighty key to healing the body.

Let's turn now and look at some ways that fasting can be used to bring health and healing to a sick body.

FOR COLDS AND FLU

Nothing is more miserable than getting a cold or flu. But did you know that the reason we suffer so much is because we do all the wrong things when we get sick? Drinking coffee and sodas and eating ice cream and pudding can make your flu or cold worse.

When you come down with a cold or flu, fast by drinking plenty of water and fresh juices, and get lots of rest. This will help your system to expel toxic materials through the mucus it creates. Let your fever burn up your infection, too. Don't rush to the doctor and take a lot of medications to halt the symptoms. Some of them are important for detoxification. However, if you have a fever over 103 degrees, you should be examined by a physician. If your fever is greater than 101 degrees and persists for longer than a few days, you should also be examined by a physician. For children, seek medical attention sooner.

Take plenty of vitamin C, garlic and herbs such as olive leaf extract, echinacea and goldenseal as a natural means to help your body's immune response.

You can overcome many infectious diseases by eliminating mucus-forming foods such as dairy products, eggs and processed grains. These grains include pancakes, cereals, doughnuts, white bread, crackers, pretzels, bagels, white rice, gravies, cakes and pies. In addition, cut out of your diet margarine, butter and other saturated, hydrogenated and processed oils.

This "Mucusless Diet Healing System" was actually developed by Professor Arnold Ehret in the early 1900s.[2]

When you are sick, don't instantly turn to antibiotics. Antibiotics can provide powerful help when you are very ill with a bacterial infection. But the overuse of antibiotics can harm you and has created resistant strains of bacteria.

Let your body's own immune system be your first defense against infections. Overusing antibiotics creates yeast overgrowth in the intestinal tract, bad (pathogenic) bacteria overgrowth in the intestinal tract and an increased risk of developing altered intestinal permeability, as well as an increased toxic burden on the liver.

Many doctors prescribe antibiotics for colds and flus that do not even respond to antibiotics. If you have had a fever of 101 degrees for a few days, go see your doctor. But don't insist on getting an antibiotic unless he or she recommends it.

FASTING FOR AUTOIMMUNE DISEASES

Autoimmune diseases are simply diseases in which the immune system attacks itself. It is a process similar to a military disaster called "friendly fire." A healthy immune system can tell the difference between normal cells and invader cells. However, in autoimmune diseases such as lupus and rheumatoid arthritis, the immune system gets confused. It actually produces antibodies that attack its own tissues. This "friendly fire" inflames the tissues. Eventually it can damage and even destroy the tissue.

Rheumatoid arthritis and lupus are autoimmune diseases that are often linked to altered intestinal permeability. This can happen when you take too many antibiotics that decrease the numbers of friendly bacteria or if your intestinal tract has been damaged by anti-inflammatory medications, aspirin or food allergies.

Another explanation for autoimmune disease is altered intestinal permeability along with poor digestion and increased consumption of meats. Most Americans eat lots of meat and other animal proteins. Meat eaters in the animal kingdom, such as lions, tigers and other carnivores, have digestive systems that secrete extremely large quantities of hydrochloric acid and enzymes. These animals also have relatively short digestive tracts.

However, humans are not so lucky. They do not produce nearly as much hydrochloric acid or digestive enzymes. In addition, our intestinal tracts are much longer. That means we aren't nearly as well equipped as lions to digest so much meat.

Combine this with the load of stress that most of us live under, stress that further reduces the amount of the digestive juices such as hydrochloric acid and pancreatic enzymes. It is no wonder we have an epidemic of bloating, gas and indigestion! And the pharmaceutical companies are making a killing.

We eat far too much protein for the amount of hydrochloric acid and digestive enzymes we have. Therefore, our stomachs and intestines can't break down the proteins into the individual amino acids as well as they should. Incompletely digested proteins called peptides are formed that can be absorbed directly into the bloodstream if you have altered intestinal permeability. Your body may form antibodies to attack these foreign substances. Once again, the body may start to attack itself; if this happens, inflammation will occur.

Too much protein, poor digestion and altered gut permeability are a recipe for autoimmune diseases such as rheumatoid arthritis and lupus. Such diseases are rare in countries where people eat mainly fruits, vegetables and whole grains such as in Japan, China and Africa. But when these same people come to the United States and adopt our diet, they begin to develop autoimmune diseases.

Fasting is one of the most effective therapies for treating autoimmune diseases. But the earlier in the course of the disease, the better.

It's extremely important to wean yourself off all medicines before you fast. Fasting allows the digestive tract to rest. It also allows the intestinal tract to heal.

Juice fasting is very beneficial in autoimmune diseases.

161

Nevertheless, some physicians have had outstanding results with water fasting. If you are going on a fast, especially a water fast, for an autoimmune disease, be sure you are carefully monitored by your physician.

If you have been taking Prednisone or other steroid drugs, it is extremely important to wean off these medicines slowly prior to fasting; be sure to watch for signs of adrenal suppression. They include severe weakness and fatigue, rapid heart rate and low blood pressure. It may take months to successfully wean off these medications.

After the fast, patients with autoimmune disease should avoid all animal proteins, dairy products and eggs. It may also be helpful to avoid wheat products, too. Instead, choose brown rice bread, rice crackers, spelt pasta and other rice products.

FASTING FOR CORONARY DISEASE

Fasting is also very effective for the treatment of heart disease and peripheral vascular disease, which usually occurs in the legs. Peripheral vascular disease is simply a buildup of plaque or atherosclerosis, usually in the arteries of the lower extremities. Renowned researcher and physician Dr. Dean Ornish proved that coronary artery disease could be reversed with a vegetarian diet, stress management and exercise.[3]

After only a year on this program, Dr. Ornish's patients had much less plaque in their arteries. If you have significant coronary artery disease or peripheral vascular disease (atherosclerosis in your legs), I recommend that you follow Dr. Ornish's complete program.

In addition, regular, periodic fasting will speed up the plaque removal process in the arteries.

While fasting, if you have significant coronary artery disease or peripheral vascular disease, you will find that your cholesterol levels will usually become more elevated on the fast. This happens because your body is in the process of breaking down plaque that is formed in the arteries, so don't be alarmed.

I always check the blood work before prescribing fasting for my patients. I'm always really encouraged when I see a dramatic elevation in cholesterol in those with coronary artery disease or peripheral vascular disease while fasting. I know that the fasting is doing its work and plaque is being broken down as atherosclerotic plaque is being removed while fasting.

HYPERTENSION

Do you have high blood pressure? One of the best ways to treat hypertension is to go on a juice fast. Before your fast, you should first attempt to get off all medications with the help of your physician and God. Increase the amount of water you drink to least two to three quarts of filtered water a day. Follow the directions for the detoxification fast outlined in this book and the instructions in my booklet *The Bible Cure for High Blood Pressure*.

FASTING FOR PSORIASIS AND ECZEMA

I have found that many of my patients with both psoriasis and eczema suffer from numerous food sensitivities. They usually have increased intestinal permeability and impaired liver detoxification, too.

It is critically important for those with both eczema and psoriasis to fast with juices to which they are not allergic. This is best done by choosing juices according to blood type or by having food allergy testing first.

If you have eczema and psoriasis, you probably also have yeast overgrowth in your intestinal tract. If you do have yeast overgrowth, prior to fasting follow a candida diet for at least three months. For more information on this topic refer to my booklet *The Bible Cure for Candida and Yeast Infections*.

If you find that you do not respond well to a juice fast, you can try a balanced rice protein fast. This product is called UltraClear Plus and can be purchased from many nutritional doctors. (See Appendix C.)

Water fasting can also be effective for psoriasis and eczema, but it must be closely monitored. If you decide to go on a water fast, supplement your fast with detoxifying teas such as dandelion and milk thistle tea.

Before going on any fast for psoriasis and eczema, follow the program for improving intestinal permeability mentioned in chapter 5. I also recommend improving liver detoxification by taking the vitamins and nutrients outlined in chapter 9.

If you have psoriasis, you probably have significant increased intestinal permeability as well as an increased toxic burden on your liver. It is critically important to repair your GI tract and detoxify your liver. It is also extremely important to avoid foods to which you are allergic.

If you don't know what foods you're allergic to, have a comprehensive food allergy test taken. I have found that many of my patients with eczema and psoriasis commonly are sensitive or allergic to dairy, wheat products, eggs, tomatoes or yeast products. This subject is discussed in more detail in my booklets *The Bible Cure for Candida and Yeast Infections* and *The Bible Cure for Allergies*.

FASTING FOR CROHN'S DISEASE AND ULCERATIVE COLITIS

Fasting is very effective for patients with both Crohn's disease and ulcerative colitis. Again, those with these diseases usually have increased intestinal permeability, toxic overload on the liver, numerous food allergies and sensitivities.

Many of my patients with Crohn's disease or ulcerative colitis are very sensitive to all dairy products, night shades (including jalapeno peppers, potatoes, tomatoes and eggplant), wheat products and often to yeast-containing products as well. These individuals are generally extremely sensitive to all forms of sugar. Simple sugars should therefore be totally eliminated from the diet.

Due to their extreme sensitivity to sugar, these people do best on either a balanced rice protein such as UltraClear Plus by Metagenics or on a water fast. Juice fasting with low-sugar vegetable juices may be effective. However, juicing can aggravate the condition and lead to worsening of diarrhea.

Once your fast is over, continue eating rice products— primarily brown rice, brown rice bread and rice crackers. Slowly reintroduce a low-protein, primarily vegetarian diet. In addition, keep a good food diary to find out what foods cause food sensitivities and avoid anything that irritates your GI tract. You may also follow the blood-type diet.

FASTING FOR ALLERGIES AND ASTHMA

Juice fasting is extremely helpful if you have both allergies and asthma. Your lungs, as well as your entire respiratory tract, are vitally important elimination organs for removing toxins. Fasting often removes many of the irritants and toxins that trigger airway hyperactivity.

Allergies—both airborne and food allergies—usually dramatically improve during a fast. This is because of the close connection between allergies and intestinal permeability and liver toxicity.

Fasting gives the digestive tract time to rest and repair. It also helps the liver detoxify. Allergic symptoms are improved and sometimes completely disappear. However, it's important to be sure that you are not allergic to any of the juices you'll be consuming. Keep a food diary while you're on your fast. Use it to help you avoid any juices that may trigger allergic symptoms or symptoms of asthma. You may have food allergy testing or simply follow the blood-type diet.

FASTING FOR TYPE 2 DIABETES

If you're a Type 2 diabetic, fasting is for you. It's extremely effective for Type 2 diabetics. However, Type 1 diabetics should not fast.

Most individuals with Type 2 diabetes also suffer from obesity. They usually have high insulin levels, but their blood cells have become resistant to the effects of insulin.

Type 2 diabetics should not fast using fruits or vegetables that have a high glycemic index, such as carrot juice. Instead, they should fast using a well-balanced, high-fiber protein supplement called UltraGlycemX by Metagenics. This can usually be prescribed by a nutritional doctor. (See Appendix C.)

It's also critically important for diabetics to be on a low glycemic diet and an aerobic exercise program. For more information on diabetes, see *The Bible Cure for Diabetes*.

"The waistline is your lifeline. It is also your dateline," according to Dr. Paul Bragg.[4] How true this statement is! Fasting is great for conquering obesity. With one-half of the population of the United States either obese or overweight, we could all do a little more fasting.[5]

Overweight individuals seem to be able to follow a strict diet for a period of time, but then they splurge and binge, eating all the wrong things. For some obese people, diet is a four-letter word. If you are one of these individuals, I recommend a healthy eating plan or a healthy lifestyle, outlined in my booklet *The Bible Cure for Weight Loss and Muscle Gain*.

Fasting for too long can actually cause you to gain weight over time, as I mentioned earlier. This is because it can lower your metabolic rate and predispose you to gain even more weight. But short, frequent juice fasts—about three days out of every month—when followed up with a healthy eating plan, can bring obesity under control quickly and easily.

Periodic short fasts help you to crucify your flesh, which is a concept I will discuss at length in the following chapters.

This crucifying of your unhealthy desires is the key to gaining control over your body, control that will last a lifetime.

When you begin to see your body as the temple of the Holy Spirit, you will gain a sense of respect for the incredible work of creative genius that your body represents. This understanding makes all the difference. Our bodies are the temple of the Holy Ghost, as we read in 1 Corinthians 3:16. The scripture goes on to say, "If anyone defiles the temple of God, God will destroy him. For the temple of God is holy, which temple you are" (v. 17).

It's written right into God's laws that we cannot destroy this temple without experiencing serious consequences. If we defile our bodies with sweets, fats, processed foods and junk foods, then one day we will probably reap a harvest in the form of degenerative disease, heart disease, arthritis, diabetes, cancer and hypertension. Whatever we sow, we will also reap.

Proverbs 23:21 says, "For the drunkard and the glutton will come to poverty." God actually puts the drunkard and the glutton in the same category. Many of us wouldn't dream of getting drunk, but we overeat frequently.

FASTING FOR BENIGN TUMORS

Undergoing the detox fasting program outlined in this book may also reduce the size of benign tumors. These include ovarian cysts, fibrocystic breast disease, lipomas, sebaceous cysts and even uterine fibroids.

If you have advanced cancer, you should not fast. But fasting will definitely help you to prevent cancer.

WHEN YOU SHOULD NOT FAST

Although fasting is a healthful lifestyle that's as old as Moses, there are many times when you should not fast.

Do not fast if you are pregnant or nursing. You should not fast if you are extremely debilitated or malnourished, including patients with AIDS, cancer, severe anemia or any severe wasting states. Do not fast before or after surgery, since it could interfere with your ability to heal after surgery.

In addition, don't fast if you have cardiac arrhythmia or congestive heart failure. Don't fast if you are struggling with mental illness, including depression, anxiety, schizophrenia and bipolar disorder. These conditions can actually get worse when you fast. Individuals with severe liver and kidney disease should not undergo a fast.

As you know, I try to wean patients off most of their medications prior to a fast. However, medications such as hormone replacement therapy and thyroid medications are safe to be take during a fast. If you are taking aspirin, anti-inflammatory medications such as ibuprofen or Aleve, Coumadin, diabetic medication, antidepressants, narcotics, chemotheraphy medications or diuretics, you should not fast.

You may continue taking very low doses of hypertensive medications during a fast as long as your physician closely monitors you. However, these should not include diuretics.

If you are taking Prednisone, you should be under a doctor's care to wean you off of this medication very slowly before fasting, or at least to the lowest effective dose. If you do not wean off Prednisone slowly, you could develop adrenal gland suppression with symptoms of rapid heart rate, low blood pressure, extreme fatigue and susceptibility to infections.

When you are being tapered off Prednisone, I also strongly recommend that you take nutritional supplements with high doses of B-complex, especially pantothenic acid, vitamin C and adrenal glandular supplements, such as Cytozyme AD by Biotics.[6] (See Appendix C.)

For any fast longer than three days, I recommend getting a checkup or physical exam by your doctor first. Have him or her do blood work and a baseline EKG. I normally perform a SMAC 24. This includes kidney function tests including creatinine and BUN, electrolytes, liver function tests, blood sugar, cholesterol and triglycerides. Along with the SMAC 24, I also perform a CBC, urinalysis and EKG. These tests should be performed prior to the fast.

During the fast, I will usually perform a SMAC 24 and UA two times a week. During each office visit, tell your doctor if you are experiencing any severe weakness, fatigue or light-headedness. Tell your doctor if you are having any irregular heartbeats. Again, if you develop an irregular heartbeat or pulse, you should be examined by your physician and should probably terminate the fast.

During a fast, it is critically important to make sure your blood potassium level remains in the normal range. Low potassium can cause dangerous arrhythmias and death. That's why it's critically important not to take diuretics on a fast. Juice fasting, however, supplies large amounts of potassium in the fresh-squeezed juices. That's why it's very unlikely that you will develop low potassium while on the juice fast. Water fasts are more likely to cause low potassium levels. Commonly, during a fast, the uric acid level is elevated. However, this is no cause for concern, since this is a normal response of the body to fasting.

If your physician cannot wean you off your medications, then it may be safer to start a partial fast. The partial fast uses fresh-squeezed fruit and vegetable juices, fresh fruit, veggies, brown rice and other cleansing foods listed earlier in this book. Eat one or two meals a day of these cleansing foods, and then have one or two meals consisting of freshly squeezed juice.

Children under the age of eighteen should not follow a strict juice fast unless they are closely monitored by a physician.

You may experience improved health by fasting with juice on your first fast. However, usually you will have to fast repeatedly to detoxify the body and achieve vibrant health.

Fasting is a healthy, biblical way to cleanse your body and soul. As you've seen, it is a wonderfully natural method of healing. But don't wait until you've become ill to begin fasting. Juice fasting is far better and more effective when you begin this lifestyle while you're still healthy. Every drink you take will be a drink to good future health!

CONCLUSION

I trust that you've discovered that one of the less-heralded wonders of your physical body is that it is an amazing, natural detoxifier. God created your body to quickly, cleanly and efficiently deal with any toxin it may encounter. But in the toxic world in which we live, it takes more than a passive approach to healthcare to live long, healthy, active, disease-free lives. It takes wisdom.

I have presented the wisdom I've gained as a medical doctor. As you do your best to apply these truths, you will reap the wonderful reward of renewed energy, vitality and health.

The power of better health through detoxification is yours. I encourage you to pursue your own good health aggressively by looking carefully at your diet and lifestyle. Your own healthy future is in your hands!

This discussion on fasting and detoxification would be incomplete if we left out the most important aspect of fasting and purification—fasting for the soul and spirit. For you see, the work of fasting doesn't stop with the physical body—fasting cleanses the total person. The greatest, most powerful work of fasting is its powerful ability to cleanse the soul. Let's look.

SECTION III—
DETOXING YOUR
WHOLE PERSON

ELEVEN

Spiritual Fasting—
What It's All About

Not only is fasting a power method of cleansing and healing the physical body, but it is also a tool for cleansing the soul. Fasting is a key to genuine and deep spirituality. Throughout the ages, those who sought to know God and desired to enter into deeper spiritual realms and giftings employed fasting as a powerful and essential tool. Found throughout the Bible, fasting was considered a key part of entering into and maintaining a powerful and spiritually dynamic walk with God.

Two words are used in the Old Testament for *fasting*. One means "to cover the mouth," and the other one means "to humble oneself." In the New Testament, the word for *fasting* literally means "not eating." The actual definition for *fasting* is "to abstain from food either partially or completely."

To perform a biblical fast you must voluntary abstain from food for a period of time–either partially or completely–for a spiritual purpose. During a spiritual fast, you deny yourself one of the most basic elements of survival, one that is loved and cherished by your body–food.

Just why would any one of us even want to consider

denying our body the cookies, cakes, ice cream, hamburgers and pizza it so much enjoys? The reason is that fasting, when accomplished through the direction and enabling of the Holy Spirit, has the power to break the gripping control of our lower nature.

Our fleshly appetite can be a ravenous animal, over-powering the spiritual man within us. When this happens it "feels" impossible to say no to a craving for sweets, fast food—or even sex, gossip or slander. These strong cravings and desires are a part of our lower, baser or more animal-like nature. The Bible calls this appetite the "flesh."

When the Spirit of God leads us to pray, but the flesh demands one more television program, we can find our-selves in the middle of an internal battle for control. Or when the bathroom scale tells us that we need to lose weight, but we find it woefully impossible not to reach for one more slice of chocolate cake or bowl of ice cream, then we are encountering this powerful grip of our flesh. It has gained prominence over our mind, will, spirit and emotions.

One way to break the power of your flesh and bring it under submission to your spirit and mind is to fast. Do you have an out-of-control temper that flares up at all the worst moments, damaging relationships with those you love? Fasting can bring that "flesh" under control.

Fasting feeds your spirit man while starving your natural man. It can soften your heart and cleanse your body to make you more receptive to God's plans. Fasting can sensitize your spirit to discern the voice and internal promptings of God's Spirit.

GAINING CONTROL

The Bible has much to say about our desires for foods that harm us rather than improve our health. For instance, Proverbs 23:1–3 says, "When thou sittest to eat with a ruler, consider diligently what is before thee: and put a knife to thy throat, if thou be a man given to appetite. Be not desirous of his dainties: for they are deceitful meat" (KJV).

In this passage, God warns us against gluttony and tells us not to be controlled by our cravings for pastries and other tempting foods that do not nourish our bodies. Verse 3 cautions not to lust after the king's "dainties." These "dainties" are delicacies, meaning they are probably high-sugar foods.

The term *flesh* in the Bible speaks about the cravings and desires of our bodies that we must conquer. These desires include the following:

1 Laziness and lethargy that keeps us from exercising

2 Cravings for sweets and fats that cause us to eat too much of all the wrong foods so that we end up piling on the extra pounds and never properly nourishing our bodies

3 Out-of-control emotions such as anger and rage that can send us into a frenzy in traffic or cause us to say hurtful things to our loved ones, which we later regret

Many more things come under the category of "flesh." Flesh can involve our thoughts, our emotions, our desires for inappropriate sex, our compulsion to binge out on sweets, our inability to stop ourselves from gossiping and much, much more. "Flesh" is nothing more than our needs, wants and cravings in their undisciplined state. This concept of the "flesh" will be important to us as I complete our discussion about detoxification.

Our flesh is ignorant. *Ignorant* is defined in Webster's Dictionary as "lacking knowledge." Hosea 4:6 says, "My people are destroyed for lack of knowledge." If your flesh rules you, you will actually be drawn to the very foods that will eventually destroy you.

THE DESTRUCTIVE POWER OF UNCONTROLLED DESIRES

It has been said that the quickest way to a man's heart is through his stomach. It was because of appetite that Eve, and later Adam, fell into sin by eating the forbidden fruit. Uncontrolled appetite for food plunged the entire human race into sin, opening the door to all of the disastrous consequences that followed, such as abuse, murder, theft and so forth. (See Genesis 3:6.)

Many generations later, Abraham's grandson Esau was also unable to gain control over his appetite for food. Esau sold his birthright, which entitled him to a position of great honor and importance, for no more than a single meal—and only a bowl of soup at that! Because of this, Esau lost the cultural privilege and blessing that came with being the first-born. Instead, Jacob, Esau's younger brother, received this prestigious title and position.

Later, Jacob—not Esau—was renamed Israel, and his twelve sons became the twelve founding tribes of a great nation. If appetite had not controlled Esau, the title and position of the blessing of Abraham and Isaac would have been his. Esau's descendants would have become the great chosen nation, rather than the offspring of Jacob.

Years later, when Israel's descendants wandered around in the hot, arid, Middle Eastern desert wilderness, the entire nation encountered the same struggle. When they were unable to get food, God supernaturally sent them manna from heaven to eat. But instead of appreciating this incredible miracle, they complained that they didn't like it. You see, it didn't satisfy their fleshly cravings. Numbers 21:5 says, "And the people spoke against God and against Moses: 'Why have you brought us up out of Egypt to die in the wilderness? For there is no food and no water, and our soul loathes this worthless bread.'"

In other words, the Israelites hated the manna, so they griped and complained and grumbled against Moses. In verses 6–7, we see the disaster that followed:

So the LORD sent fiery serpents among the
people, and they bit the people; and many of
the people of Israel died. Therefore the people
came to Moses, and said, "We have sinned, for
we have spoken against the LORD and against
you; pray to the LORD that He take away the
serpents from us." So Moses prayed for the
people.

In this particular instance Moses prayed, and God healed these grumblers. But this wasn't the first time that such a thing occurred. Their uncontrolled appetites had gotten them into big trouble before. Let's look.

Now the mixed multitude who were among
them yielded to intense craving; so the children
of Israel also wept again and said: "Who will
give us meat to eat? We remember the fish
which we ate freely in Egypt, the cucumbers,
the melons, the leeks, the onions, and the
garlic; but now our whole being is dried up;
there is nothing at all except this manna before
our eyes."
—NUMBERS 11:4–6

As you can see, the Israelites caved in to their uncontrolled appetites and mumbled, groaned and complained loudly that they wanted to enjoy the same food they had in Egypt. Here's what happened next:

Now a wind went out from the LORD, and it
brought quail from the sea and left them
fluttering near the camp . . . And the people

stayed up all that day, all night, and all the
next day, and gathered the quail (he who
gathered least gathered ten homers [a homer
was about 10½ bushels; ten homers, 105
bushels]); and they spread them out for
themselves all around about the camp. But
while the meat was still between their teeth,
before it was chewed, the wrath of the LORD
was aroused against the people, and the LORD
struck the people with a very great plague.
—NUMBERS 11:31–33

Whether or not these birds were diseased, we don't really know. We do know that out-of-control fleshly cravings got these people into big trouble.

We must be very careful not to dismiss these stories as irrelevant. These accounts are extremely relevant to our own lives, for we are made of the same stuff of which these ancient wanderers were made. The uncontrolled appetite of our lower natures is just as dangerous to our own health and well-being as it was to theirs.

FLESHLY CRAVINGS

Let's investigate the lower nature a little further. Just what does it crave? These verses in 1 John spell it out:

Do not love the world or the things in the
world. If anyone loves the world, the love of
the Father is not in him. For all that is in the
world—the lust of the flesh, the lust of the
eyes, and the pride of life—is not of the Father
but is of the world.
—1 JOHN 2:15–16

What the Bible calls "the lust of the flesh" includes the following cravings:

○ Desiring excessive amounts of the wrong foods such as sweets, fats and meats; a glutton (Prov. 23:1–3)

○ Sex outside of marriage

○ Impure and ungodly desires

○ Thinking about and desiring inappropriate sex

○ Compulsive and obsessive desires for things other than God

○ Anger and angry outbursts when you don't get your own way

○ Creating strife by undermining people, criticizing and gossiping

○ Sedition or rebellion, or simply demanding that those over you do it your way, or else you'll find a way to get what you want regardless

○ Murders, which can include destroying those who get in your way, abortions

○ Drunkenness and reveling (Gal. 5:19–21)

What the Bible calls "the lust of the eyes" is really nothing more than an uncontrolled desire for sex outside of marriage or a longing for what belongs to other people, such as positions, power, riches, beauty, possessions and strength. The lust of the eyes causes us to lift ourselves above others and feel smug and self-righteous.

FASTING TO CONTROL THE LOWER NATURE

Since we are all born with the same lower nature, what can we do? Fasting is a powerful tool to subdue the strength of our flesh. Fasting can help us control the lower nature's cravings, bringing our flesh under subjection to our minds and spirits.

THE WAR BETWEEN
YOUR FLESH AND SPIRIT

The key to our spirituality is yielding to the Holy Spirit. Our fleshly, carnal nature opposes God's Spirit and cannot yield. Romans 8:7–8 says, "Because the carnal mind is enmity against God; for it is not subject to the law of God, nor indeed can be. So then, those who are in the flesh cannot please God." This means that it is impossible to walk in the power of the Holy Spirit and live in the fleshly, carnal nature.

The Bible encourages us to walk in the presence and power of the Spirit as an anecdote for living in the flesh. In Galatians 5:16–17 Paul says, "I say then: Walk in the Spirit, and you shall not fulfill the lust of the flesh. For the flesh lusts against the Spirit, and the Spirit against the flesh; and these are contrary to one another, so that you do not do the things that you wish."

As long as our fleshly, carnal nature controls us, we will be unable to do the will of the Holy Spirit because it is in direct opposition to His will.

The carnal, unrenewed mind of the flesh is controlled and dominated by the thinking and reasoning of our intellects. Emotions also control and dominate this lower nature, which means that your feelings and desires control you. In addition to that, the carnal nature is also controlled by the five senses of taste, smell, sight, feeling and hearing.

But we are not without hope, for the power of God is released through the Holy Spirit who works in us. Ephesians 3:20 tells us, "Now to Him who is able to do exceedingly abundantly above all that we ask or think, according to the power that works in us . . . " That power at work in us is the power of the Holy Spirit. However, it cannot be released in us if we are walking in the flesh.

The promise of Acts 1:8, that we will be divinely empowered by the Holy Spirit to become witnesses of God's power and love, cannot be realized by the lower, carnal nature. Jesus taught that we must crucify the flesh by taking up our own cross, just as He took up His cross. If we don't, we will be unable to yield to the Holy Spirit's power and will be fully controlled by the power of the flesh.

It's only as we live our lives in vital connection with the living Christ that we become able to crucify the lusts of the flesh and live and walk in the higher nature of the Holy Spirit within.

This process of crucifying the flesh must be accomplished daily through prayer, renewing the mind by regularly reading the Word of God and by watching every word that comes out of our mouths. All of these things are like the hammers, pickaxes, drills and machinery that operate at the rock quarry of your hardened flesh. In this effort, fasting is the dynamite that makes all of the other efforts easier and more effective.

ABIDING IN THE WORD OF GOD

The Word of God says, "Walk in the Spirit and you shall not fulfill the lust of the flesh" (Gal. 5:16). This verse suggests that what you focus upon will empower your thoughts. If you focus upon the Spirit of God through prayer and fill your mind with the Word of God, your thoughts will be filled with the power of God to resist negative, poisonous emotions and attitudes.

Our minds must be renewed so that we will be able to walk in the Spirit and not fulfill the desires of the flesh. This renewing of the mind occurs as our thoughts are filled with the powerful, living Word of God. But if our minds are always thinking upon negatives such as jealousy, envy, strife, unforgiveness or what makes us angry, or upon things we don't have but want, on someone who has hurt us or caused us harm and on what we dislike, then our minds and thoughts are carnal or inspired by our lower nature. When we fill our minds with God's words and thoughts through the Bible and prayer, we feed and strengthen our higher nature, which was designed to serve God.

This is the secret to overcoming temptation—even the temptation of dangerous emotions.

ABIDING IN CHRISTLIKE SPEECH

Often our mouths get us into more trouble than anything else. They may well be our greatest weapons of destruction. In fact, James 3:6 says, "And the tongue is a fire, a world of iniquity. The tongue is so set among our members that it defiles the whole body, and sets on fire the course of nature; and it is set on fire by hell." What we say often releases the destructive power of our lower natures into the atmosphere or into individual lives and relationships. How often have we all wished we could take back some of the things we've said?

What you say has enormous spiritual, emotional and physical power. Proverbs 18:21 says, "Death and life are in the power of the tongue." Your words actually have the power to heal or kill, to strengthen or wound, to unite or divide. Controlling your words is extremely important. Here are some scriptures about the tongue to recite every time you are tempted to slip and say something you know you'll regret:

- "Out of the abundance of the heart the mouth speaks" (Matt. 12:34).

- "For every idle word men may speak, they will give account of it in the day of judgment" (Matt. 12:36).

- "Let no corrupt word proceed out of your mouth" (Eph. 4:29).

Paul talked about his victory over the carnal nature in 1 Corinthians 9:25–27. Paul said he "disciplined" his body and made it his slave. He accomplished this in part through fasting. The apostle tells us in Romans 13:14 to make no provision for the flesh to gratify its desires. In Colossians 3:5 Paul tells us to "mortify" our members (KJV). In 1 Corinthians 9:25 Paul says to bring the body into subjection.

We are to crucify the flesh according to Galatians 2:20 and Romans 6:6. In 1 Peter 2:11 we are told to abstain from fleshly lust. We must decide: Is the body the master, or is the Holy Spirit the master? The body makes a wonderful servant but a very poor master.

Fasting brings the carnal nature into subjection so that the body becomes the servant and the Spirit becomes the master, allowing us to walk in the power of the Holy Spirit.

In addition to helping us conquer the seemingly insurmountable power of the flesh, fasting has many other powerful spiritual applications.

THE WHY OF SPIRITUAL FASTING

So why should we fast? What does denying ourselves our favorite foods actually do for us?

BUILDS GODLY CHARACTER

For starters, fasting builds character. By enabling us to surrender our lives to God in greater measure, we find more control over our tongues, our minds, our attitudes, our emotions, our bodies and all our fleshly desires. Fasting also helps us to submit our spirits to God completely so that He can use them for His purposes.

It really is possible to be led by the Spirit of God and not ruled by fleshly desires. However, even though many Christians have invited the power of the Holy Spirit into their lives, they continue to be led about by the insatiable appetites of the flesh. They live their lives pursuing whatever gratifies the cravings of the lower nature or their own selfish motives instead of the purposes of God. Many are good people who actually would like to live on a much higher plane of existence, but they just don't know how.

Fasting allows us to die to the appetites of the lower nature, to the lusts of the flesh. It gives us the ability to build up character and integrity by allowing the Spirit of God to operate through us. The only real way to build godly character and genuine integrity into our inner man is by spending time in the presence of God.

LOOSES CHAINS OF BONDAGE

Do you struggle with addictions or addictive behaviors? Sometimes addictions can even show up in our personalities rather than through debilitating behaviors such as alcoholism. For instance, perhaps you've never been an alcoholic, but when you get into a room filled with people you have an obsessive need to be constantly talking or running everything and everyone in sight. An exaggerated need to control others or to control circumstances and situations can be just as much of a bondage as a drug addiction.

Bondages come in all shapes, colors, types and sizes. So don't be too quick to dismiss the notion that you may have some bondages in your own life. Most of us growing up and living in this very imperfect world end up with some bondages. Those who do not are by far the very rare exception—if they even exist at all.

Do you have bondages in your life? Or do you have close loved ones who are bound by addictive personalities and behaviors? Fasting is critically important if you have children who need to be set free from drugs and alcohol, homosexuality, pornography or who have been caught up in the throes of rebellion. Fasting can be extremely helpful when you are praying for a loved one's salvation. Is there strife in your home or workplace? Fasting can begin to break any spiritual stronghold so that peace and civility can return.

Isaiah 58:6 says that fasting is to "loose the bonds of wickedness, to undo the heavy burdens, and to let the oppressed go free, and that you break every yoke."

HUMBLES OURSELVES

Although the lower nature can seem amazingly powerful, fasting humbles it. Humbling the flesh is required if we want to live a clean, godly life.

Matthew 18:4 says, "Therefore whoever humbles himself as this little child is the greatest in the kingdom of heaven." First Peter 5:6 says, "Therefore humble yourselves under the mighty hand of God, that He may exalt you in due time." James 4:10 says, "Humble yourselves in the sight of the Lord, and He will lift you up." Matthew 23:12 says, "And whoever exalts himself will be humbled, and he who humbles himself will be exalted."

One of the key reasons that fasting gets God's attention is that it is a key to humility. Fasting humbles our flesh, which finds favor with God. James 4:6 says, "God resists the proud, but gives grace to the humble." In other words, the humility that can be obtained through spiritual fasting opens the door to God's grace and favor.

God doesn't make us humble. He has left that responsibility up to us. We humble ourselves before God with fasting and prayer, as individuals and even as a nation.

FASTING FOR SPIRITUAL HEALING, GLORY AND REFRESHING

America needs to be healed. Our children need to be healed from the spirits of rebellion, drugs, alcohol, revelry, homosexuality, sexual lusts and perversion. Our land needs to be healed from the shedding of innocent blood because of the millions of abortions occurring every year. Our culture needs to be healed from the selfishness and self-centeredness that have consumed us, causing us to constantly crave more things, more money and more power. We are a people desperately in need of spiritual healing.

As we have seen, fasting is a powerful tool for spiritual healing, whether for a nation as a whole, for cities, for families or for individuals.

We are promised in God's Word that if we fast and pray as a group that an awesome spiritual healing can take place. Let's look:

If My people who are called by my name will humble themselves, and pray and seek My face, and turn from their wicked ways, then I will hear from heaven, and will forgive their sin and heal their land.
—2 CHRONICLES 7:14

Again we see that attitude and motive are as important as fasting itself. Even though our culture rewards pride, God does the exact opposite. He rewards the self-imposed humility obtained through fasting. Humbling ourselves helps us to shift our focus away from the pleasures, concerns and demands of our lives here on earth and to focus upon the things above—God and His priorities.

Such humble fasting has created a force that has won wars, stayed judgment and saved cities and countries. Humble fasting before God is awesomely powerful and can turn an entire nation around.

FINDING THE PRESENCE OF GOD

Have you ever desired to experience God's presence? Fasting can bring the healing and refreshing presence of God into an individual life and into the life of a family or even a nation. Too many of us let natural things absorb our time and energy when we could be enjoying the glorious realm of God's Spirit.

After Moses fasted for forty days, he was swept up into an

entirely new place in God's Spirit. He received the Ten Commandments and became the lawgiver of Israel. After Jesus had fasted for forty days, the Holy Spirit empowered His life, and His ministry of healing and preaching was launched.

You too can receive the touch of God's glory upon your own life, just as Jesus and Moses did, through fasting and prayer. The kind of prayer that simply makes long lists of requests to God is not enough. You must enter into the realm of the Holy Spirit through worship, reading God's Word and listening to God's voice as well as making requests.

Moses experienced the same hunger for more of God that you may be experiencing right now. He prayed that God might reveal Himself to him, although no man could actually look at God and live. His request is found in Exodus 33. The Lord then instructed him,

And the LORD said, "Here is a place by Me,
and you shall stand on the rock. So it shall be,
while My glory passes by, that I will put you in
the cleft of the rock, and will cover you with
My hand while I pass by. Then I will take away
My hand, and you shall see My back; but My
face shall not be seen."
—Exodus 33:21–23

In other words, Moses got a glance of the glory of the back of God. Exodus 34:29–32 says:

Now it was so, when Moses came down from
Mount Sinai (and the two tablets of the
Testimony were in Moses' hand when he came
down from the mountain), that Moses did not
know that the skin of his face shone while he
talked with Him. So when Aaron and all the
children of Israel saw Moses, behold, the skin
of his face shone, and they were afraid to come

187

near him. Then Moses called to them, and
Aaron and all the rulers of the congregation
returned to him; and Moses talked with them.
Afterward all the children of Israel came near,
and he gave them as commandments all that
the LORD had spoken with him on Mount Sinai.

Moses' encounter with God was so powerful that he actually shone with God's glory, and the people, blinded by the
light that was on him, shrank back in fear. Moses' dynamic
experience with God went much further than merely impact-
ing his own life. The touch of God he received dramatically
impacted the entire nation.

The radiant glow shining on his face was so bright that
Moses covered his face with a veil to keep from blinding
those around him. Verse 33 says, "And when Moses had fin-
ished speaking with them, he put a veil on his face."

Fasting allowed Moses to enter such a depth of God's presence that the very glory of God came upon him and radiated
to everyone nearby. Fasting created such a sense of God's
power and presence upon him that God's glory overflowed.

Fasting enables us to touch the world around us with
God's love and power. Fasting can be a tool to access God's
power to affect our children, our extended families, our cities
and even the world. Acts 1:8 says, "But you shall receive
power when the Holy Spirit has come upon you; and you
shall be witnesses to Me in Jerusalem, and in all Judea and
Samaria, and to the end of the earth."

In fact, it was with fasting that the apostles in the first
century sent out their missionaries to proclaim the message
of Christ. Acts 13:2–3 says, "As they ministered to the Lord
and fasted, the Holy Spirit said, 'Now separate to Me
Barnabas and Saul for the work to which I have called them.'
Then, having fasted and prayed, and laid hands on them,
they sent them away."

FASTING DELIVERS US FROM ERROR

When you are making critical decisions such as choosing your mate, changing a job, deciding to move or other major life-impacting decisions, you need God's divine guidance to be sure you are not holding onto opinions or other judgments that are in error.

The problem with error is that when we're in it, we think we're right. That's why we need divine guidance for life's major decisions.

The Bible promises that the Holy Spirit is ready and willing to provide that guidance when you ask. John 16:13–14 says, "However, when He, the Spirit of truth, has come, He will guide you into all truth; for He will not speak on His own authority, but whatever He hears He will speak; and He will tell you things to come."

The apostle Paul received this kind of guidance in Acts 9 after meeting Jesus Christ on the road to Damascus. Before he became a believer, the apostle actually was very hostile to the church of Jesus Christ. A wave of persecution swept through the early church, and Paul was one of its leaders. While erroneously following his own best judgment, Jesus Christ appeared to him and he fell to the earth.

Blinded by the light of the risen Savior, the Lord told him to visit a particular house. He had to be led by hand for three days, during which time he fasted, nether eating nor drinking.

Paul genuinely believed that he was serving God by persecuting Christians until he heard Christ's voice saying, "Why are you persecuting me?"

But when Paul asked, "Who are You, Lord?"

The reply was . . . "I am Jesus."

Fasting will free you from your own misjudgments and allow the light of Christ's truth to shine clearly.

There are times in all of our lives when we are being led around by our own misjudgments and desires, and we don't even know it. Regular fasting can protect us from the blindness of our own opinions and desires.

Fasting will help us to be led by the Spirit instead of being led by faulty judgments. Paul was a good man, but his faulty judgments caused him to actually fight against God instead of fighting for Him. It's tragic that we humans can be so blind—but we can! That's why spiritual fasting is so very important.

FASTING FOR HEALING

Fasting is also a powerful tool for healing and restoration. Here's what the Bible says about it:

Then your light shall break forth like the morning, your healing shall spring forth speedily, and your righteousness shall go before you; the glory of the LORD shall be your rear guard.
—ISAIAH 58:8

Not only does fasting break the chains of wickedness, lift heavy burdens and free the oppressed, but it also brings back your health.

THE WHEN OF SPIRITUAL FASTING

It's important to fast for the right motive, but I'll bet you didn't know that it's equally important NOT to fast at certain times. The disciples of Jesus learned this truth.

**The disciples of John and of the Pharisees were fasting. Then they came and said to Him, "Why do the disciples of John and of the Pharisees fast, but Your disciples do not fast?"
And Jesus said to them, "Can the friends of the bridegroom fast while the bridegroom is**

with them? As long as they have the bridegroom with them they cannot fast. But the
days will come when the bridegroom will be
taken away from them, and then they will fast
in those days."
—MARK 2:18–20

When Jesus was walking with them through the hills of Galilee, teaching them and praying with them, fasting was inappropriate. It was neither the time nor the season to fast. Rather, His presence brought a season of rejoicing and feasting. However, after Jesus ascended into heaven, the disciples were expected to fast.

In Mark 2:20, Jesus said, "They will fast in those days."

Still, we don't actually read about the disciples fasting until the Book of Acts. In Acts 13:1–3 the church fasted together as they were guided by the Holy Spirit or had a need.

After the followers of Christ began fasting, they had rich teaching provided by the Master from which to draw. Jesus had taught them all about motives and even about appearance during times of fasting. In Matthew 6:17–18, Jesus said, "But you, when you fast, anoint your head and wash your face, so that you do not appear to men to be fasting, but to your Father who is in the secret place; and your Father who sees in secret will reward you openly."

Jesus did not say "if" you fast, but "when" you fast. He assumes that fasting will be a normal part of spiritual life once He, the Bridegroom, is gone.

So then, when should we fast? Always fast as the Holy Spirit leads. In other words, just as Jesus was led into the wilderness to fast and pray, we should also be led by the Spirit into times and seasons of fasting. The New Testament never lays down strict rules regarding fasting; therefore, we should never impose strict rules upon others or ourselves.

REGULARLY SCHEDULED FASTS

Even though most spiritual leaders were called to a fasted lifestyle, throughout time many have been called to fast for regularly scheduled times. Let's investigate.

We know that the Jewish leaders fasted regularly, usually twice a week. The Bible mentions their regular fasts in Luke 18:11–12.

The Pharisee stood and prayed thus with himself, "God, I thank You that I am not like other men—extortioners, unjust, adulterers, or even as this tax collector. I fast twice a week; I give tithes of all that I possess."

The *Didache* was a Christian manual on the practices of the church that was written in the second century. The *Didache* actually ordered regular weekly fasts on both Wednesdays and Fridays. The writers of this document said, "Let not your fast be with hypocrites, for they fast on Mondays and Thursdays, but do you fast on Wednesdays and Fridays."[1] By ordering regular fasts, the *Didache* was doing just as it criticized the Pharisees for doing—it was promoting legalism.

Later the Roman Catholic Church set aside Fridays as its fast day. No Catholic Christian was permitted to eat meat on Fridays. Even Martin Luther, the leader of the Protestant movement, promoted fasting. However, he insisted that fasting be voluntary and private.

John Wesley, on the other hand, recommended that Christians fast on the two week days that were mentioned in the *Didache*—Wednesdays and Fridays. Wesley refused to ordain an individual in the Methodist ministry if he didn't fast on those days.

Other great men of God fasted regularly also, men such as Andrew Murray, Charles Finney, Charles Spurgeon and John G. Lake.

A commitment to regular fasting is another powerful way to enjoy the benefits of a fasted lifestyle. For today's disciples who regularly minister to hurting individuals, fasting is a mighty tool of spiritual empowerment.

As we've seen, fasting is very important in spiritual life. But we've also seen that not all fasting is helpful. Legalistic fasting earned the Pharisee in Luke no brownie points with God. The reasons for which we should take up spiritual fasting are always totally selfless.

As we've seen, God is most concerned with our motives for fasting. Jesus too was far more concerned with the motives behind fasting than with how long or how often we fast. Motive is everything when it comes to spiritual fasting.

IN CONCLUSION

Do you desire to experience the mighty power and supernatural presence of God in your life? I trust that by now you have realized that it may require more from you than a simple prayer. To go deeper into spiritual things you may have to humble yourself by combining fasting with your prayer. Do you desire for God to change seemingly insurmountable circumstances in a loved one's life or in your family or workplace? Fasting can empower your prayers and break the strongest bondage and oppression.

Spiritual fasting is a mighty key that, when accomplished with the right motives, produces powerfully dynamic results.

Let's turn now and look at how fasting was used in just these very ways by great men and women throughout history.

TWELVE

Spiritual Fasting Throughout the Bible

The Bible says that when we fast or stop eating for spiritual purposes, then God will feed us something better than food. Isaiah 58:14 says He will feed us with "with the heritage of Jacob." What that means is that fasting will give us a place among other great spiritual men and women throughout history.

This is an incredible promise, for many great men and women have rocked nations and shaken kingdoms. Walking in their footsteps is a genuine privilege.

Let's turn now and look at some of these spiritual giants and examine their powerful spiritual fasts. They are named for the great spiritual leaders who used them to make their world better and to rise above the human, fleshly condition.

Jesus Himself employed fasting to conquer Satan.

Let's investigate the fast of Jesus. The story begins when Jesus was baptized by John the Baptist. In Luke 3:21–22, the Bible states, "Jesus also was baptized; and while He prayed, the heaven was opened. And the Holy Spirit descended in bodily form like a dove upon Him, and a voice came from heaven which said, 'You are My beloved Son; in You I am well pleased.'"

This is the first of two major experiences Jesus had before entering public ministry. In this experience, the Holy Spirit descended upon Him in a visible form. If Kodak cameras had been available back then, no doubt someone would have snapped pictures of this powerful phenomenon. Even so, this incredible sign from heaven did not launch Christ's ministry. After the Holy Spirit came down upon Him, He was led by the Spirit into the wilderness to fast and pray (Matt. 4:1).

For forty days Christ ate nothing. After this extended fast, Luke 4:14 says, "Then Jesus returned in the power of the Spirit to Galilee, and the news of Him went out through all the surrounding region."

Later, Jesus would sit among the people and teach three disciplines in the Sermon on the Mount. They include prayer, giving and fasting—and He placed all three on the same level. Many believers feel it is their duty to pray and give but seldom feel the same need to fast. But Jesus didn't say, "If you fast . . . " He said "When you fast . . . " (See Matthew 6:17–18.)

Jesus didn't begin His ministry until He had fasted for forty days. Jesus was first baptized. Then the Holy Spirit descended on Him, and afterward He was full of the Spirit. The Holy Spirit led Him into the desert, and after His fast, He returned in the power of the Holy Spirit. This was when His mighty ministry was launched, a ministry of great miracles, signs and wonders. All of this took place as a result of fasting.

Interestingly, Jesus told us that we too would do these works and even greater works because He went to the Father. (See John 14:12.) I truly believe that we will see these greater works as we learn and practice the great spiritual discipline of fasting.

If Jesus Christ felt the need to fast, how much more should we? Fasting can be accomplished by an individual, a group of people or by an entire nation. When the Jews came together each year on the Day of Atonement for a day of corporate fasting, the results were powerful. Let's take a look.

CORPORATE FASTING FOR FORGIVENESS OF SINS

Historically, God's people were commanded to fast once a year. On the Day of Atonement, all Israel came before God in corporate fasting and repentance. (See Leviticus 16:29–34; 23:26–32.)

The Day of Atonement was considered the single most sacred day of the entire religious year, a day in which everyone in the entire nation stopped everything he was doing, refused to eat and sought God's forgiveness for all the sins committed that year.

Leviticus 16:29 tells us:

This shall be a statue forever to you: In the seventh month, on the tenth day of the month, you shall afflict your souls, and do no work at all.

Another translation says, "You must deny yourselves and not do any work" (NIV). It goes on to say, "Because on this day atonement will be made for you, to cleanse you. Then, before the LORD, you will be clean from all your sins. It is a sabbath of rest, and you must deny yourselves; it is a lasting ordinance" (vv. 30–31, NIV).

Since the day this statute was given, for the past thirty-five hundred years, Jews have honored and observed Yom Kippur, or the Day of Atonement, as a solemn day of fasting. This fast day was mentioned in the New Testament. As Paul journeyed to Rome, "much time had been lost, and sailing had already become dangerous because by now it was after the Fast [which was the Day of Atonement]" (Acts 27:9, NIV).

The Day of Atonement usually fell at the end of September or the beginning of October. The fasting of this special day was part of the humility and repentance necessary for atonement to be given by God. On this day, the high priest actually laid hands on a goat and spoke out the people's sins. When he was through, he released the goat into the desert or the wilderness. The blood of another goat was then sprinkled in the holy of holies in a solemn act. Through this ceremony, the sins of the people were cleansed.

The Day of Atonement was always on a Sabbath day. During Jesus' lifetime, the Jews observed about twenty-two different spiritual fasts, including the Day of Atonement fast.

Not only was fasting used to cleanse the sins of an entire nation, corporate fasting was used by the Jews also to seek protection and deliverance when their enemies tried to destroy them.

THE ESTHER FAST—FOR PROTECTION, DELIVERANCE AND DIVINE FAVOR

Esther was a beautiful, young Hebrew girl living in Persia during Israel's captivity. This lovely woman was chosen as queen over all the other young women in the entire nation. The prime minister of Persia was Haman, an evil man who hated the Jews.

Haman succeeded in passing a law of genocide to kill all the Jews. Therefore, Queen Esther decided to risk going before the king to try and save her people. According to the laws, if anyone, even the queen, requested an uninvited audience with the king, that person could be killed.

Faced with the danger to her people and the danger to Esther herself, the queen called a fast. The Bible says:

Go, gather together all the Jews who are in
Susa, and fast for me. Do not eat or drink for
three days, night or day. I and my maids will

fast as you do. When this is done, I will go to
the king, even though it is against the law. And
if I perish, I perish.
—ESTHER 4:16, NIV

Esther went before the king dressed, not in sackcloth and
ashes, but with her royal robes. She invited Haman and the
king to a banquet she had prepared, and the king accepted.
However, later that night the king could not sleep. He had
his royal diary brought in, and as the diary was being read,
he learned that Esther's cousin Mordecai had saved his life.
The king's heart had already been turned toward Esther
because of the people's corporate fast.

When Haman entered the court to speak with the king
about another matter, the king asked Haman this question:
"'What should be done for the man the king delights to
honor?' Now Haman thought to himself, 'Who is there that
the king would rather honor than me?'" (Esther 6:6, NIV).

Haman answered the king with these words:

Have them bring a royal robe the king has
worn and a horse the king has ridden, one
with a royal crest placed on its head. Then let
the robe and horse be entrusted to one of the
king's most noble princes. Let them robe the
man the king delights to honor, and lead him
on the horse through the city streets, proclaim-
ing before him, "This is what is done for the
man the king delights to honor!"
—ESTHER 6:8–9, NIV

Just before this happened, Haman had prepared gallows
to hang Mordecai. But instead of hanging him, Haman was
forced to parade him with great tribute throughout the city.
Then Esther informed the king that Haman had issued the
decree to have the Jewish people exterminated. The king
entered as Haman was reaching for the queen to beg for

mercy. It looked to the king as if Haman was attempting to assault his wife sexually. The story ends with Haman being hanged on the gallows that were prepared for Mordecai.

The three days of corporate fasting called by Esther turned the situation completely around in a mighty display of supernatural favor and spiritual power.

The three-day Esther fast is for protection, deliverance and divine favor, and it reveals the power of corporate fasting to move the hand of God mightily and to change the hearts of men. This fast opens up even those whose hearts are bitterly hardened against God and can help turn hurting individuals back to God.

Let's turn now and look at the fast of another great leader whose spiritual fast significantly impacted a nation's history.

THE EZRA FAST— FOR DIRECTION AND PROTECTION

For centuries the nation of Jews was held in captivity by the nation of Persia. When freedom finally came, Ezra, a priest, was given permission by Cyrus, the king of Persia, to return to Jerusalem to rebuild the magnificent Jerusalem temple.

The trip to Jerusalem was very dangerous. Ezra needed protection to lead the great caravan of thousands of defenseless Jews back to their home city. He was ashamed to ask the king for an escort of soldiers because he had bragged about God's protection for all who worship Him. Many of the travelers actually had become wealthy in captivity, and so Ezra was responsible for safely transporting their treasures and other belongings as well.

Ezra 8:21 says, "I proclaimed a fast, so that we might humble ourselves before our God and ask him for a safe journey for us and our children, with all our possessions" (NIV). They fasted for the protection, security and direction from God.

The journeyers returned to Israel in safety with all of their possessions intact. Once again, the Bible reports powerful spiritual results were obtained through fasting.

Although corporate fasting was common, individual fasts were even more so. Elijah was another spiritual giant of the Bible who understood the power of fasting for affecting the outcome of great spiritual battles. The Elijah fast is undertaken during times of intense spiritual conflict.

THE ELIJAH FAST— TO COMBAT SPIRITUAL ENEMIES

Elijah had just won the greatest victory of his life over four hundred fifty prophets of Baal. He actually had called fire down from heaven and then had all of those demonically inspired prophets of Baal killed. Queen Jezebel, who had given these prophets a place of authority, responded in an angry frenzy, threatening to murder Elijah by the very next day.

Thrown into a state of terror, depression and despondency, Elijah ran for his life. He didn't stop running until he was about a day's journey away in the wilderness, where he sat down to rest under a juniper tree. It seems clear that Elijah realized that he lacked what it took to battle what was coming against him. In 1 Kings 19:5–8, we read:

Then as he lay and slept under a broom [juniper] tree, suddenly an angel touched him, and said to him, "Arise and eat." Then he looked, and there by his head was a cake baked on coals, and a jar of water. So he ate and drank, and lay down again. And the angel of the LORD came back the second time, and touched him, and said, "Arise and eat, because the journey is too great for you." So he arose, and ate and drank; and he went in the strength of that food forty days and forty nights as far as Horeb, the mountain of God.

In this account, Jezebel represents the evil forces that can come against God's own. The Bible says, "For our struggle is not against flesh and blood, but against the rulers, against the authorities, against the powers of this dark world and against the spiritual forces of evil in the heavenly realms" (Eph. 6:12, NIV). Confronted with the rage of evil forces, Elijah responded with fasting.

Elijah didn't eat or drink, and the power of the terror, despondency and depression that had assailed his mind and overwhelmed his emotions was broken.

We all have faced overwhelming situations that terrify us, paralyze us and place us in emotional and mental bondage. There are even times in which we feel as if the very forces of hell are raining down on us.

Nonetheless, we don't have to be become paralyzed or bound by a yoke of anxiety, depression and fear. Just as with Elijah, God has provided fasting as a powerful weapon to combat the spiritual forces that attack our minds and emotions.

Isaiah 58:6 says, "Is this not the fast I have chosen: to loose the bonds of wickedness, to undo the heavy burdens, to let the oppressed go free, and that you break every yoke?" Yokes are devices for joining two oxen together. When you are yoked with depression, you become bound or united to it as a heavy burden that you must carry.

Yokes of bondage include negative attitudes such as depression, despondency, fear and anxiety. But don't go on a forty-day fast as Elijah did without a special word from God, no matter how heavy your yoke. Even then, your physician must closely monitor such a lengthy fast. Also, never go on a fast without drinking adequate amounts of water on a daily basis.

Both Elijah and Moses went on a supernatural fast in which they ingested neither food nor water. Jesus, however, went on a forty-day fast and drank water, but ate no food. Interestingly, on the Mount of Transfiguration, Elijah and Moses—the two men who had fasted for forty days without food or water—were there with Jesus. (See Matthew 17:2–3.) All three who stood on the Mount together had undergone a forty-day fast.

Fasting finds great favor in God's sight because of its ability to break the control of the flesh. Daniel was another great spiritual leader whose fasting brought about powerful results. Let's take a look at the Daniel fast for overcoming the flesh.

THE DANIEL FAST— TO OVERCOME THE FLESH

Daniel and three other Hebrew youths, Shadrach, Meshach and Abednego, were Jews in captivity, but in the kingdom of Babylon. They were greatly favored for their purity, and they were well educated and extremely gifted both mentally and spiritually.

When these four young men were captured and taken into the king's palace to educate them in the ways of the Chaldeans, Daniel 1:5 states, "The king assigned them a daily amount of food and wine from the king's table" (NIV). He planned to keep them on his own rich diet of meats, fats, sugary pastries and wine for three years. At the end of the three years they would be presented to the king.

However, verse 8 says, "But Daniel resolved not to defile himself with the royal food and wine" (NIV). In other words, Daniel rejected the rich, temptingly delicious meats, wine and pastries of the royal court, perhaps because they did not meet the requirements of Jewish dietary laws or because these youths may have taken vows against drinking alcohol.

So Daniel made a request of the prince of the eunuchs. Verse 12 says, "Please test your servants for ten days: give us nothing but vegetables to eat and water to drink" (NIV). The King James version uses the word *pulse*. "Pulse" consisted *of vegetables and grains, wheat, barley, rye, peas, beans and lentils.*

Daniel and the three other Hebrew youths lived a fasted

life for three years on the vegetarian diet of pulse while learning and studying in the king's court, and God honored their
partial fast. We're told in verse 15, "At the end of the ten
days they looked healthier and better nourished then any of
the young men who are the royal food" (NIV).

God tremendously favored their decision to fast and
granted them favor, wisdom and insight far above anyone
around them. In verses 18–20 (NIV) we read:

At the end of the time set by the king to bring
them in, the chief official presented them to
Nebuchadnezzar. The king talked with them,
and he found none equal to Daniel, Hananiah,
Mishael and Azariah; so they entered the king's
service. In every matter of wisdom and understanding about which the king questioned them,
he found them ten times better than all the
magicians and enchanters in his whole kingdom.

Daniel knew what was healthy to eat, and he purposed in
his heart that he would not defile himself. The Daniel fast
eliminates rich foods such as meats, pastries, cakes, pies, cookies, alcohol and any other food that is tempting to the flesh.

Today, people are so bound to their flesh that they often
cannot go one meal without eating some form of meat,
something sweet, fatty or some other type of rich food. We
must crucify our flesh daily and take up our cross and follow
Christ. (See Matthew 16:24.) What better way to crucify our
flesh than to follow Daniel's fasted lifestyle?

THE SECOND DANIEL FAST— FOR SPIRITUAL BREAKTHROUGHS

We find a second fast of Daniel in which he took in nothing
but water. Let's look.

Daniel 9:3 says, "Then I set my face toward the Lord God
to make request by prayer and supplications, with fasting,

sackcloth, and ashes." When the Jews fasted with sackcloth and ashes, it was never a partial fast, but a total fast with complete abstinence from food.

Again, during a season of special prayer when Daniel desperately needed revelation from God, he fasted. Daniel 10:2–3 says, "In those days I, Daniel, was mourning three full weeks. I ate no pleasant bread, no meat or wine came into my mouth, nor did I anoint myself at all, till three whole weeks were fulfilled."

Many people believe that this was a partial fast or a diet. However, many scholars believe it was a total fast. During this time of fasting, Daniel had great visions from heaven, along with an incredible angelic visitation.

This time of fasting reveals some astonishing insights into the spiritual realm and how it works. Once again, we see fasting as a dynamic agent of powerful spiritual warfare. It seems that the great ruling angel, Gabriel, was attempting to get a message to Daniel from the moment Daniel started praying. However, the account paints a picture of a great spiritual struggle encountered by this angelic being that was broken as Daniel fasted.

The mighty, shining heavenly ruler spoke to Daniel. "Since the first day that you set your mind to gain understanding and to humble yourself before your God, your words were heard, and I have come in response to them. But the prince of the Persian kingdom resisted me twenty-one days" (Dan. 10:12–13, NIV).

The angel spoke of powerful, spiritual demonic princes and great, high-ranking angels sent to withstand these beings. The fascinating thing about this passage is the place it gives to fasting and prayer. It was because of Daniel's three-week fast that the great angel was able to breakthrough the dark opposition and meet with Daniel to provide the mighty revelation he was seeking.

This astonishing passage suggests that fasting is extremely

important when we need a breakthrough. In addition to that, it also suggests that we must never give up when we are seeking God.

Throughout the Bible, those who believed in God and wanted to develop spiritually sought God through the discipline of fasting. The disciples of Jesus were among them also.

THE DISCIPLES' FAST— FOR EMPOWERED MINISTRY

When the disciples who traveled with Jesus were sent out to begin ministering on their own, they encountered some unexpected resistance to the healing power of God. When the disciples were powerless to heal a young boy, the child's father approached Jesus.

The father's request is recorded in Matthew 17:15.

Lord, have mercy on my son, for he is an epileptic and suffers severely; for he often falls into the fire and often into the water.

Apparently the father didn't understand that his son was actually gripped by a demonic force. Although most cases of epilepsy have physical causes, this particular case did not.

In Matthew 17:16, we see that the father had taken his son to the disciples, but they were powerless to respond. Many of our own youth, teens and young adults are bound with alcohol, drugs, nicotine, sexual desire, a spirit of revelry and partying, homosexuality, satanism, witchcraft, palm reading and other dangerous strongholds. Unfortunately, some of these young people are Christians, but they are still bound with fear, anger, bitterness, resentment, unforgiveness, jealousy, strife, envy and many other deadly emotions.

How can our youth be bound with these strongholds and yet profess to know Christ? Here's how. They may have had their sins forgiven, and they may have professed Christ as their Savior, but they have never had the spiritual chains of wickedness broken off of them. Isaiah 58:6 says, "Is this not the fast that I have chosen: to loose the bonds of wickedness, to undo the heavy burdens, to let the oppressed go free, and that you break every yoke?"

The disciples' fast breaks yokes, or breaks mental, spiritual and emotional bondages, and sets people free. If you are a mother or father with a son or daughter in rebellion, bound with homosexuality, sexual perversion, sexual desire, drugs, alcohol or any other stronghold, Jesus Christ can set them free by applying the principles of the fast of the disciples.

In Matthew 17:17–21, it's clear that Jesus expected the disciples to exercise enough faith to heal the demonized boy. He rebuked them by saying:

"O faithless and perverse generation, how long shall I be with you? How long shall I bear with you? Bring him here to Me." And Jesus rebuked the demon, and it came out of him; and the child was cured from that very hour.

Then the disciples came to Jesus privately and said, "Why could we not cast it out?"

So Jesus said to them, "Because of your unbelief; for assuredly, I say to you, if you have faith as a mustard seed, you will say to this mountain, 'Move from here to there,' and it will move; and nothing will be impossible for you. However, this kind does not go out except by prayer and fasting."

This boy's seizures were the result of a demonic stronghold that required fasting and prayer to break. Although demonic strongholds are created by sin, it doesn't necessary follow that everyone who sins is bound by evil forces. But if sin seems impossible to resist, causing an individual to repeatedly fall back into destructive behaviors, then a stronghold may be involved. Strongholds include alcoholism, drug addition, sexual addictions, compulsive lying, stealing or any other strongly compulsive behavior.

To overcome a stronghold, first you must recognize it for what it is—a powerful way in which dark forces have attempted to control you. Next, it is important to avoid people and situations that link you to that stronghold. For example, if you are an alcoholic, stay away from bars and avoid your old drinking buddies.

It's also important to watch what you say. Your words hold great power. Try to speak words that will bring faith and life, not depression and hopelessness. In other words, when you are tempted, don't say, "This thing is bigger than me. I'll never get free." Instead, speak the powerful Word of God, *If the Son of God has set me free, then I am free indeed!* (See John 8:36.)

Join your faith together with the faith of other believers. Have them pray for you and with you. Visit and share your feelings with those who will help you to stay focused and strong.

If you have never asked Christ to come into your life, I encourage you to do so. There is great freedom in the power and fellowship of the Holy Spirit. Salvation is no farther away than the whisper of a prayer. Why not invite Jesus Christ into your heart this very minute? Simply bow your head and pray this prayer:

Dear Jesus, I repent for all of my sins. I repent for the sins that have brought bondage and fear into my life and into the lives of others. I thank You for dying on a cross for me so that I might be free. I receive Your forgiveness right now. Jesus, come into my heart, for I give my life to You. In Jesus' name, amen.

If you have just prayed this prayer, freedom and release are yours. Christ has forgiven your sins and entered your heart. Accept it by faith, which is nothing more than choosing to believe God. And by the way, welcome to the family!

Continue to build up your faith through Bible reading,

praying and speaking the Word of God. Now, if you have received Christ, prayed and done everything else we've discussed and still continue to struggle against a stronghold, you may need to do some fasting to break its power over you.

Interestingly, when Jesus encountered those who were demon possessed, He never attempted to heal them. Rather, He cast out the demon. Another example of Jesus' dealings with demonic strongholds can be seen in Mark 5:1–16.

In Mark 5:8–9, Christ spoke to the stronghold. He said:

"Come out of the man, unclean spirit!" Then He asked him, What is your name?" And he answered, saying, "My name is Legion; for we are many."

Unfortunately, today we treat most addictions and diseases with drugs, when the actual cause may be a satanic stronghold. An individual receiving such treatments will never be truly healed until the stronghold is dealt with. This usually requires prayer and fasting.

The Bible describes the disciples' fast to break strongholds in Isaiah 58:6 where God gives us the reasons for fasting. As we read earlier, it says, "Is this not the fast that I have chosen: to loose the bonds of wickedness, to undo the heavy burdens, to let the oppressed go free, and that you break every yoke?"

Other great ministers in the Bible fasted. For instance, Moses fasted for forty days, as recorded in Exodus 24:18. Interestingly, Moses fasted for forty days at least two other times. (See Exodus 34:28; Deuteronomy 9:18.)

I strongly discourage you from ever fasting without drinking water. Water is absolutely essential for life, and we can only live about four days without water. Moses and Elijah had a supernatural fast, since they neither consumed food nor water. In addition, never fast beyond three days without being under the care of a nutritional physician.

Some other great ministers who fasted in the Bible include King David, the great prophet Samuel, the apostle Paul and John the Baptist.

LIVING A FASTED LIFE

Many great ministers with special callings in the Bible actually went beyond fasting. They lived a fasted lifestyle.

John the Baptist was one of these individuals who lived his entire life in a partially fasted state. We see this lifestyle described in Matthew 3:4.

And his food was locusts and wild honey.

John the Baptist was a Nazirite. He was called to a Nazirite vow and a fasted life before he was even born. That call is recorded in Luke.

For he will be great in the sight of the Lord,
and shall drink neither wine nor strong drink.
He will also be filled with the Holy Spirit,
even from his mother's womb.
–LUKE 1:15

John the Baptist lived a fasted life that included eating locusts and wild honey for his protein. Otherwise, he was a total vegetarian, most likely supplementing his diet of honey-coated bugs with fruits, vegetables and some grains.

Another well-known Nazirite was Samson. He kept a life-long fast from wine and alcoholic beverages and from touching anything that had died. Therefore, Samson was probably a vegetarian, too. In addition to that, Samson vowed never to cut his hair. (See Judges 13:4–5.)

These faithful men lived in a deeper level of devotion and separation to God than most people today even understand. Instead of feeding his flesh, John the Baptist hungered for the things of God. Jesus said in Matthew 5:6, "Blessed are those who hunger and thirst for righteousness, for they shall be filled."

By living fasted lives, John the Baptist and Samson were empowered to speak a word of prophecy and deliverance to their generations. John the Baptist stormed the countryside, preparing the crowds for the coming of Christ.

The fasted lives of these individuals signaled that they were born for a great and special purpose. Their lives were not their own, but were to be lived in complete devotion to God.

Are you interested in going on a spiritual fast? Do you seek to influence your nation, city, workplace or family? Would you like to break through the strength of your flesh or the power of a particular bondage? I trust you've discovered some powerful insights into fasting through this list of biblical spiritual fasts. I encourage you to select the fast that most suits your particular spiritual goals. Appendix B is a practical fasting workbook that will help you to get focused and to begin.

CONCLUSION

I trust that you've discovered that fasting is a powerful tool for health, cleansing, corporate strength and spiritual empowerment. The Bible gives fasting an ancient position of honor, a place beside other dynamic principles for health and spiritual growth.

Fasting is a privilege, and it is a biblical key to cleansing that will bless your life with the gift of health, healing, renewed vitality, longevity and deeper spirituality.

As you begin to undergo periodic juice fasts for detoxification, I encourage you to first commit that time to God for spiritual cleansing and renewal. Once you become accustomed to fasting for two or three days, you may choose to increase that time a little. Learn to devote increasing portions of that time to Bible reading, prayer and journaling for personal and spiritual growth. At times you may even choose to commit your fast times to even higher purposes, such as fasting for issues of national cleansing and healing.

As you develop a life of fasting and prayer, you will find that God will feed you with the heritage of Jacob. You will walk in the footsteps of great men and women who have gone before us—men and women who increased in purity of body, mind and spirit, and who touched heaven with their prayers and nations with their passion.

—Don Colbert, M.D.

Other Solutions for Toxic Relief

While it's vitally important to detoxify your body, there are other measures you can take to live free from the effects of this toxic planet. Here are some additional helpful solutions to help you stay healthy.

AIR POLLUTION

Avoid heavy smog and gasoline fumes. If you are waiting for a taxi at the airport and the air outside is full of fumes from traffic and buses, then go inside to wait. Don't stand around at a bus station in fume-filled areas behind the buses. Never sit in heavy traffic with your window open, and if you are following a motorist whose car emits a cloud of nauseating fumes, take another route, if necessary, to get away from those dangerous emissions, which are high in carbon monoxide, hydrocarbons and many other chemical pollutants.

Never jog or run alongside a busy highway where your lungs can be absorbing high amounts of carbon monoxide, hydrocarbons and other toxins.

SICK BUILDING SYNDROME

You can minimize sick building syndrome in your home by choosing less toxic carpets or installing hardwood floors or tile floors. Use less toxic paints. Never buy or use furniture made of pressed wood or particleboard. Instead, choose hardwood or metal furniture. Select drapes made of cotton instead of fabrics that have been treated with formaldehyde.

Plants have a wonderful practical use, as well as creating an attractive environment. Plants actually take in carbon dioxide and many other dangerous gasses and give off clean, pure oxygen. If you suspect that the office building in which you work is sick, surround your work place with plants. Spider plants, philodendrons, Boston ferns and English ivy are all easy-to-grow, hardy indoor plants. Best yet, they tend to be excellent natural air purifiers.

BACTERIA, MOLD AND YEAST

Minimize your exposure to mold spores and dust mites by keeping the heating and air conditioning ducts in your home clean. Set up a schedule for periodic cleaning, and stick with it.

In addition, lower the relative humidity in your home to less than 45 percent. This will discourage the growth of mold and dust mites. Take special note of the rooms in your home that tend to be most damp, such as the bathroom and laundry room.

If you live in a very humid climate, you may want to consider purchasing a dehumidifier for your home.

Use an air purifier such as a hepa filter or ionizer air filter to remove chemicals and toxins in the air. Open the windows and doors in your home during the day in order to get fresh air. It is also a good idea to open the windows or doors in your office in order to get fresh air and to dilute some of the toxic air. It is even better to have a ceiling fan on with a window open since there is even a better exchange for outside air.

However, be sure and dust the top of the fan periodically.

Purchase some air-purifying plants such as spider plants, English ivy or Boston ferns, to name a few.

PESTICIDE POLLUTION

One of the most important ways you can reduce your exposure to pesticides is to stop having your home sprayed. Try more natural methods of bug control, such as sprinkling cupboards and closets with boric acid.

Avoid the use of air fresheners or air deodorizers. Try more natural air fresheners, such as a pot of fragrant flowers on your dining room table. Better yet, open your windows on cool mornings and evenings to air out your home. If you have a window that catches a regular breeze, try planting fragrant flowers such as jasmine nearby. Aromatic plants can refresh your home with a lovely, natural scent while at the same time providing natural air purifiers and fresh oxygen.

Ask everyone to take their shoes off before coming inside from outdoors. This is a major way that pesticides are brought in. House dust can accumulate large amounts of pesticides that have been tracked in from outside, and vacuuming every day just tends to send them into the air, making the situation even worse. It's much simpler to cultivate the habit of having everyone remove their shoes.

SECONDHAND SMOKE

Do not allow smoking in your home. Avoid areas where secondhand smoke is present.

TOXINS IN OUR WATER

A shower filter such as a charcoal or KDF shower filter (see Appendix C) is effective in removing chlorine and, thus, in preventing the formation of trihalomethanes or THM.

Your Fasting Journal

This special fasting journal will help you grow and develop as a total person—body mind and spirit—as you learn to fast. Set aside time for reflecting, journaling, prayer and Bible reading during your fast period. Before long, you will begin to touch the dynamic benefits of fasting for the cleansing and healing of the heart, mind, body and spirit.

Each day's journal page includes a place for you to record your prayers, prayer requests, thoughts and insights.

This program calls for repeated periods of two to three fasts. Each time you fast, come back to the journal and take up where you left off. If you fast for longer periods, then work through the daily journal pages throughout the term of your fast.

BEFORE YOU BEGIN . . .

Before you begin this time of fasting, prayer, personal reflection and spiritual growth, here are some considerations that will help you to prepare your heart.

During your fast, meditate on Scripture throughout the day, read the Bible and ask the Holy Spirit, your Teacher, to give you divine revelation.

Listen to Bible teaching tapes while you're driving, at work or at home to help you stay focused on God's Word.

Pray as often as possible, or do as the Scripture says and pray without ceasing. Set aside certain specific times for prayer and journaling. Here are some pointers that will also help:

○ Take time to be quiet before the Lord and listen to the voice of the Spirit.

○ Record in your journal what the Holy Spirit is revealing to you.

○ Write down prayer requests.

○ Write down revelation and insights given to you during the fast.

○ Write down praise reports.

○ Write down any dreams and pray for the interpretation of them.

Before you start, it's important to set the boundaries of your fast. Determine what type of fast you will go on. Check <✔> the boxes below that identify fast or fasts you will be implementing.

❏ A partial fast, as in Daniel

❏ A water fast (do not go over three days unless followed by a doctor)

❏ A fruit and vegetable juice fast (as discussed in this book)

❏ A fast with a powdered protein supplement (such as UltraClear Plus or UltraGlycemX)

❑ A word fast (a refusal to speak any words that hurt, injure or cause fear, doubt, anger strife, shame or guilt)

❑ A fast from media, TV, Internet and radio in order to listen to the Bible on tape or listen to teaching tapes instead

❑ A fast from harsh, critical words at home (This fast will help you as a mother or father to use language that is courteous, kind and uplifting to children. It will help you as a husband or wife to speak only encouraging, uplifing words to your spouse.)

❑ A fast from gossip (Are you surrounded by gossip, criticism and negativity at work or with a social group? This fast helps you gain control over such deadly, toxic social environments. Simply refuse to gossip about anyone and refuse to listen to any gossip.)

Now that you've set your parameters, it's time to get started. I pray that these special days of cleansing and healing will be some of the most rewarding days of your entire life. I pray that you will experience renewed health, energy and vitality. In addition, I pray that your soul and spirit will be refreshed and renewed as well.

So, let's get started.

DAY ONE

PREREQUISITES TO FASTING

You will not fast as you do this day, to make your voice heard on high. Is it a fast that I have chosen?
—Isaiah 58:4–5

1 What are your purposes for fasting?

❑ To set free a child on drugs or alcohol

❑ To set free a child in rebellion

❑ For the salvation of a child, friend or family member

❑ To break a spirit of strife over a home business or church

❑ To break an addictive relationship

❑ Other _____

2 Are you fasting for divine guidance and revelation for yourself or a loved one?

❑ In deciding whom to marry

❑ In deciding what job or what field of study to choose

❑ In deciding where to move

❑ For deciding what type of work God would have you to do

❑ For promotion in your job, as Joseph was promoted from Potiphar's house to second in command of all of Egypt behind Pharaoh

❑ For wisdom to understand the need for that promotion

❑ Other _____

3 Commitment: Write a statement of commitment to God about why you are fasting and what you hope will be accomplished during this special time.

_____

_____

_____

_____

_____

4 Dedication: Write a prayer of dedication, devoting this fast time to God and to His purposes in your life.

_____

_____

_____

_____

_____

_____

DAY TWO

REPENTANCE AND RECONCILIATION

You shall cry, and He will say, "Here I am." If you take away the yoke from your midst, the pointing of the finger, and speaking wickedness.

–ISAIAH 58:9

Fasting is a way to help you to enter into God's presence where you can minister to Him through praise, worship and thanksgiving. Here are some steps to follow to help you enter into God's presence.

1 First, identify and confess all sin before the fast and repent. Also, do so during the fast.

Write a list of any sin you may have in your life.

_____

_____

_____

2 Now, write a prayer confessing and repenting to God for those sins.

_____

_____

_____

_____

_____

_____

_____

3 Ask the Holy Spirit to identify any strongholds such as anger, fear, hatred, envy, jealousy, bitterness, unforgiveness, rejection, shame, guilt, blame, abandonment, grief or inadequacies that are separating you from God. Ask the Holy Spirit to help you forgive yourself and anyone else who has wronged you and to break the stronghold.

_____

_____

_____

4 The Holy Spirit may prompt you to seek reconciliation and restoration from someone who has wronged you. Ask God to show you any person or people to whom you must go and seek reconciliation. What are their names?

_____

_____

_____

5 Write out a prayer from your heart asking God for help to truly forgive and bless ALL others.

_____

_____

_____

_____

_____

DAY THREE

A PROMISE OF REFRESHING

The LORD will guide you continually, and satisfy your soul in drought, and strengthen your bones; you shall be like a watered garden, and like a spring of water, whose waters do not fail.
—ISAIAH 58:11

The Bible promises mental, physical and spiritual refreshing during fasting.

1 Write about your need for refreshing.

_____

_____

_____

_____

_____

2 Write a prayer asking God to refresh specific areas in your life.

_____

_____

_____

_____

_____

_____

RELEASING BURDENS

Is this not the fast that I have chosen: to loose the bonds of wickedness, to undo the heavy burdens?
—Isaiah 58:6

Fasting will also set you free from burdens.

1 This means a fast will enable you to be set free from burdens such as:

❑ Financial burdens

❑ The stresses of everyday life

❑ Chronic illness of yourself or a loved one

❑ Legal problems, including lawsuits, bankruptcies, foreclosures or incarceration

❑ The burden of taxes

❑ Dealing with difficult neighbors, coworkers or family members

2 Write in your journal about your circumstances.

_____

_____

3 Write out a prayer asking for God's help and giving your burdens to God. Thank Him for it.

_____

_____

_____

DAY FIVE

FASTING FOR HEALING

Your healing shall spring forth speedily.
—Isaiah 58:8

One of these burdens is sickness. You may also fast for a longstanding or recurrent illness of yourself or a loved one.

1 List the loved ones and their needs for whom you're fasting.

_____

_____

_____

_____

_____

_____

2 Write out a prayer asking God to heal your loved ones.

_____

_____

_____

_____

_____

_____

_____

DAY SIX

A RELEASE OF GOD'S POWER

And your righteousness shall go before you.
The glory of the LORD shall be your rear
guard.
—ISAIAH 58:8

Fasting helps to release the power of the Holy Spirit in
one's life.

1 Do you want to see God's power released in your
life? Write about it.

_____

_____

_____

_____

_____

2 Write a prayer asking God for more power in your
life to lead more to the Lord.

_____

_____

_____

_____

_____

_____

DAY SEVEN

PROTECTION AND SAFETY

... to loose the bonds of wickedness.
—Isaiah 58:6

Fasting will provide you with protection, safety and deliverance.

1 What circumstances do you need God's help with?

❑ Protection and deliverance from domestic violence

❑ Safety from physical harm

❑ Protection of your home, your finances and business

❑ For safety and protection of your children in school, day care or any other public place

2 The Book of Esther shows divine protection of the children of Israel by the fast of Esther and Mordecai. Read through the Book of Esther today.

3 When you are fasting you should be communing with God during the fast. This is how you will receive God's protection and His deliverance. Here are some other promises you can claim for yourself during this period of fasting.

He who dwells in the secret place of the Most High shall abide under the shadow of the Almighty. I will say of the Lord, "He is my refuge and my fortress; my God in Him I will trust." Surely He shall deliver you from the snare of the fowler.
—Psalm 91:1–3

4 Write a prayer thanking God for His protection.

_____

_____

_____

_____

_____

_____

_____

_____

_____

_____

DAY EIGHT

EXPECTING THE BENEFITS OF FASTING

Then you shall call, and the LORD will
answer; you shall cry, and He will say, "Here
I am."
—ISAIAH 58:9

While you are fasting, you should also be expecting.
Expect God to do wonderful things in your life while
you are on your fast. Study the list of benefits of fasting
from the Bible.

1 Fasting builds character and integrity. "But I discipline my body and bring it into subjection, lest, when I have preached to others, I myself should become disqualified" (1 Cor. 9:27). Fasting helps to break the carnal nature, which allows us to be led by the Spirit and, therefore, to walk in integrity.

2 Fasting brings the flesh under subjection. Isaiah 58:6 says fasting will loose the bands of wickedness.

3 So many people are controlled by the lusts of the flesh. Romans 13:14 warns us to make no provision for the flesh to gratify its desires. In 1 Peter 2:11, we are instructed to abstain from the passions of the flesh.

4 Fasting allows us to loose the bands of wickedness, which are the strongholds of the flesh.

5 Fasting enables us to seek the presence of God. Isaiah 58:9, 11 says, "Then you shall call, and the LORD will answer. You shall cry, and He will say, 'Here I am' . . . The LORD will guide you continually, and satisfy your soul in drought, and strengthen your bones. You shall be like a watered garden, and like a spring of water, whose waters do not fail."

6 Fasting enables you to preach with power and authority. Read Acts 1:8 and Acts 13:3.

7 Fasting will allow spiritual revival—first in your own family, and then in your church, in your city and eventually in the whole nation. Read 2 Chronicles 7:14.

8 Write out a prayer thanking God for all of the many benefits He is giving to you during your fast.

_____

_____

_____

_____

_____

_____

_____

BEING LED BY THE SPIRIT DURING FASTING

The Lord will guide you continually.
—ISAIAH 58:11

To realize all of the benefits of fasting, you must be led by the Spirit during this special time. Spend some time reading about fasting and about the Spirit of God in the Bible.

1 Fasting should be led by the Spirit to receive spiritual benefits. Luke 4:1–2 explains how Jesus fasted. He was led by the Spirit and was full of the Spirit.

2 Jesus endorsed fasting in Matthew 6:1–18 and actually said, "When you fast . . . " He did not say, "If you fast . . . " However, when you fast at the Spirit's leading, do it with specific purposes in mind.

What Spirit-led purposes do you have for fasting today?

_____

_____

_____

_____

_____

3 The church fasted as the Spirit guided them or as they had need. Read Acts 13:1–3.

4 The Spirit led Jesus into the wilderness. The Lord also led Moses. In Exodus 24:12, the Lord told him to come up into the mountain. There Moses remained with God for forty days and forty nights without food or water. Read about these accounts.

Describe how you feel God led you to start fasting?

_____

_____

You should fast when a need or situation in life calls for it. If you have a great need to hear from the Lord for direction and guidance, or any of the other above reasons, the Spirit will usually lead one on a fast.

5 Write out a prayer of thanks to God for leading you to fast.

_____

_____

_____

_____

_____

_____

_____

DAY TEN
YOUR MOTIVATION FOR FASTING

Indeed you fast for strife and debate.
—Isaiah 58:4

Spend some time reflecting about your own motives for fasting. Are your motives pure? Reflect on the questions below.

1 The Pharisees demonstrated spiritual pride when they fasted. Are your motives to impress others?

_____

_____

_____

_____

2 Fasting is worthless if it becomes a ritual or routine. Has fasting become just a routine part of your life?

_____

_____

_____

_____

3 Fasting can cause self-righteousness, which exalts a person in his own eyes and in the eyes of others. Do you fast to gain the approval of those who see you fasting?

_____

_____

_____

4 Will you get personal gain or benefit from fasting, or is it for the Lord's benefit?

_____

_____

_____

_____

5 We should fast for the benefit of others, not merely for ourselves. Will your fast benefit others?

_____

_____

_____

_____

6 Write a prayer asking God to forgive you for any wrong motives for fasting and to fill your heart and mind with motives that are pure.

_____

_____

_____

_____

_____

_____

REFLECTIONS

REFLECTIONS

REFLECTIONS

Product Information

T hroughout this book you may have noticed that various products have been mentioned. For your convenience, here's a listing of these products and how to purchase them:

○ Biotics (including friendly bacteria with FOS, request BioDolphilus-FOS. For adrenal support, request Cytozyme AD) 1-800-874-7318

○ Divine Health Green Superfood, Divine Health Whole Food Multivitamin, Divine Health Buffered Vitamin C, Divine Health Basic Antioxidant, Divine Health Advanced Antioxidant www.drcolbert.com or 1-407-331-7007

○ Filters Charcoal and KDF Online Store: FilterDirect.com

○ Great Smokies Diagnostic Lab for 1) Comprehensive Digestive Stool Analysis with Parasitology, 2) Intestinal Permeability Testing 3) Food Allergy Testing. Web address: www.gsdl.com

○ Longevity Plus Friendly Bacteria and FOS, request Inuflora and Primal Defense call 1-800-580-PLUS

○ Metagenics (including UltraClear Plus and Ultra GlycemX) Call 1-800-647-6100

○ Vita-Mix Mixer—Web address: www.Vita-Mix.com

○ Wellness Water filters: 1-888-667-8082, ext. 214

○ To locate a nutritional doctor call ACAM 1-800-LEAD-OUT (1-800-532-3688)

NOTES

Introduction

1. Source obtained from the Internet: Leading Causes of Death in the United States, 1994; www.ers.usda.gov/publications/aib 70.

Chapter 1
Our Toxic Earth

1. Jacqueline Krohn, *Natural Detoxification* (Vancouver, BC: Hartley & Marks Publishers, Inc., 1996).
2. C. C. Patterson, "Contaminated and Natural Lead Environments of Man," *Archives of Environmental Health* 11 (1965):344.
3. E. Cranton, *By-Passing By-Pass* (Troutdale, VA: Medex Publishers, 1996), 97.
4. Source obtained from the Internet: EPA Office of Environmental Information, www.epa.gov/triexplorer/chemical.htm.
5. *Harrison's Principles of Internal Medicine,* 12th edition (New York: McGraw-Hill, 1991.
6. 22nd Annual Surgeon General's Report on Smoking and Health.
7. G. T. Sterling, et al, "Health effects of phenoxy herbicides," *Scandinavian Journal of Work Environmental Health* 12 (1986): 161–173.
8. Rachel Carson, *Silent Spring* (Boston MA: Houghton, Mifflin, 1962).
9. Krohn, *Natural Detoxification.*
10. John Lee et al., *What Your Doctor May Not Tell You About Premenopause* (New York: Waner Books, 1999).
11. J. B. Weston, and E. Richter, *The Israeli Breast Cancer Anomaly* (New York: Academy of Sciences, 1990), 269–279.
12. J. Beasley, et al, "The Kellogg Report: the impact of nutrition, environment and lifestyle on the health of Americans," New York Institute of Health Policy and Practice, The Baird College Center, 1989.

13. Theo Colborn, *Our Stolen Future* (New York: Penguin Group, 1997), 150–152.
14. Ibid.

Chapter 3
Overnourished While Starving?

1. Source obtained from the Internet: http://www.ers.usda.gov/publications/aib750.
2. Don Colbert, M.D., *What You Don't Know May Be Killing You* (Lake Mary, FL: Siloam Press, 2000), 108.
3. Source obtained from the Internet: W. Batalion, Americans for Safe Food, www.cgs.com.
4. C. H. Barrows, "Nutritional Aging: the time has come to move from laboratory research to clinical studied," *Geriatrics* 32 (1977): 39.
5. Paul Bragg, *The Miracle of Fasting* (Santa Barbara, CA: Health Science, 1983).
6. C. Ruckner, et al., *The Seventh-Day Adventist Diet* (New York: Random House, 1991).
7. B. Jensen, *Tissue Cleansing Through Bowel Management* (Escondido, CA: Bernard Jensen Enterprises, 1981).
8. Ibid.

Chapter 5
The Joy of Juice

1. Source obtained from the Internet: http://www.ams.usda.gov/fu//.
2. J. Selhub, et al., *American Medical Association*, 270 (1993): 2693–2726.
3. R. G. Ziegler, "A review of epidemiologic evidence that carotenoids reduce the risk of cancer," *JNutr* 119 (1989): 116–122.
4. E. Giovannucci, et al., "Tomatoes, lycopene and prostate cancer," *Proc Soc Esp Biol* 218 (1998): 129–139.
5. "Caret Trial," by the National Cancer Institute, n.p.
6. K. A. Steinmetz, et al., "Vegetables, Fruit and Cancer," Two Mechanism, *Canc Causes Control*, 2 (1991) : 427–442.
7. American Cancer Society "Nutrition and prevention," (New York: American Cancer Society, 1984).
8. D. Ahn, et al, "The effects of dietary ellagic acid on rat hepatic and esophageal mucosal cytochrome P450 and Phase 2 enzymes," *Carcinogenesis* 17 (1996): 821–828.
9. S. A. Glynn et al., "Folate and cancer: a review of the literature," *New England Journal of Medicine* (1998): 1176–1178.

Chapter 6
Dr. C's Detox Fast

1. Peter J. D'Adamo, M.D., *Eat Right for Your Blood Type* (New York: Putnam's Sons, 1997).
2. Ibid., 334.
3. Ibid., 335.
4. Ibid., 336.
5. Ibid., 333.
6. Elson Haas, M.D., *Staying Healthy With Nutrition* (Berleley, CA: Celestial Arts Pub., 1992).

Chapter 9
"Eliminate the Negative"

1. Don Colbert, M.D., *The Bible Cure for Heartburn and Indigestion* (Lake Mary: FL Siloam Press, 1999), 3.
2. D. Burkett and H. Trowell, *Western Diseases and Their Emergence and Prevention* (Cambridge, MA: Harvard University Press, 1981).
3. Ibid.
4. Colbert, *The Bible Cure for Heartburn and Indigestion*, 4.
5. K. J. Pienta, et al., "Inhibition of spontaneous metastasis in rat prostate cancer model by oral administration of modified citrus pectin," *Journal of the Nutritional Cancer Institute*, 87 (1995): 348–353.

Chapter 10
Finding Healing Through Fasting

1. George H. Malkmus, *Why Christians Get Sick* (Shippensburg, PA: Destiny Image Publishers, 1995), 19, 103.
2. Arnold Ehret, *Muscusless Diet and Healing System* (Beaumont, CA: Ehret Literature, 1972).
3. Dean Ornish, et al., "Can lifestyle changes reverse coronary heart disease?" *Lancet* 336 (1990): 129–133.
4. Bragg, *The Miracle of Fasting*.
5. H. L. Steward, *Sugar Busters* (New York: Ballantine Books, 1998), 246.
6. Don Colbert, M.D., *The Bible Cure for Chronic Fatigue and Fibromyalgia* (Lake Mary: FL Siloam Press, 2000).

Chapter 11
Spiritual Fasting—What It's All About

1. J. B. Lightfoot, *The Apostolic Fathers*, edited and completed by J. R. Harner (Grand Rapids, MI: Baker Books Press, 1956).

Pick up these other Siloam Press
books by Dr. Colbert:

Walking in Divine Health
What You Don't Know May Be Killing You
The Bible Cure® Booklet Series

The Bible Cure for ADD and Hyperactivity
The Bible Cure for Allergies
The Bible Cure for Arthritis
The Bible Cure for Cancer
The Bible Cure for Candida and Yeast Infection
The Bible Cure for Chronic Fatigue and Fibromyalgia
The Bible Cure for Depression and Anxiety
The Bible Cure for Diabetes
The Bible Cure for Headaches
The Bible Cure for Heart Disease
The Bible Cure for Heartburn and Indigestion
The Bible Cure for High Blood Pressure
The Bible Cure for Irritable Bowel Syndrome
The Bible Cure for Memory Loss
The Bible Cure for Menopause
The Bible Cure for Osteoporosis
The Bible Cure for Prostate Disorders
The Bible Cure for PMS and Mood Swings
The Bible Cure for Sleep Disorders
The Bible Cure for Stress
The Bible Cure for Weight Loss and Muscle Gain

SILOAM PRESS
A part of Strang Communications Company
600 Rinehart Road
Lake Mary, FL 32746
(800) 599-5750

Don Colbert, M.D., was born in Tupelo, Mississippi. He attended Oral Roberts School of Medicine in Tulsa, Oklahoma, where he received a bachelor of science degree in biology in addition to his degree in medicine. Dr. Colbert completed his internship and residency with Florida Hospital in Orlando, Florida. He is board certified in family practice and has received extensive training in nutritional medicine.

To have Dr. Don and Mary Colbert hold
a health seminar at your church or town,
for other speaking engagements or if you would
like more information about
Divine Health Nutritional Products®,
you may contact:

DON COLBERT, M.D.

1908 Boothe Circle
Longwood, FL 32750
Telephone: 407-331-7007

Dr. Colbert's website is
www.drcolbert.com.

DISCLAIMER: Dr. Colbert and the staff of Divine Health Wellness Center are prohibited from addressing a patient's medical condition by phone, facsimile or e-mail. Please refer questions related to your medical condition to your own primary care physician.